SIMPLE CHANGES
TO
END
CHRONIC
PAIN

NANCY LEE SHAW

Editor: Anne DeMarsay, Voices Into Print
Book Design and Production: Dash Parham
Cover Design: Glendon Haddix, Streetlight Graphics
Illustrations: Keala Weinstock
Printed in the United States of America

www.createspace.com

Dedication

I am dedicating this book to two very influential women in my life: my mother, Marie Jackson Shaw, who by example and word encouraged me, and quietly challenged me, to strive for the best in all that I wanted to achieve; and Janet G. Travell, M.D., my mentor and guide in the field of myofascial trigger point pain and dysfunction. Her challenge was to never give up and to allow myself to accept the time and energy required to solve the pain puzzles that were presented to me. To both, I am forever indebted.

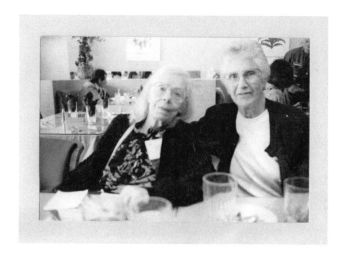

Acknowledgments

My thanks first to those physicians and practitioners who have been involved over the years in the development of the field of myofascial pain and dysfunction at a time when it seemed a difficult concept to embrace.

Special gratitude goes to my sister, Gail, for her many prayers, cards, and telephone calls to remind me to take my time and to enjoy what I was doing. Warm gratitude also goes to my close friends, Sigrid and TAG, who encouraged me to write this book and gave me the space and support to follow it through to the end. Thank you to the many friends for their invaluable understanding, along with their taking the time to read and reread the manuscript as it developed. Their presence gave me the ongoing focus necessary to always see that the end was, indeed, in sight. Throughout the years, family and friends were my most important and fun-loving support system. Of course, their scheduled breaks for me were just what I also needed.

Special thanks to Dash Parham, my graphic artist with unending patience, without whom this project would not have been accomplished, to Dixie Vereen for using her unique skills to take basic muscle drawings and making them pieces of art, and to Anne DeMarsay, my editor, for stepping in and pulling things together in such an expert way. To Keala Weinstock, thank you for the excellent stretch illustrations throughout the book.

I would be remiss not to offer a big thank-you to all the patients who allowed me to use their photographs to teach the principles put forth in this book. I am grateful to all my patients who have been a constant source of challenge to me to grow in the knowledge and understanding of pain and its elimination.

Contents

Foreword

M uscle is a "stepchild" in modern medicine. Somehow, no medical specialty has adopted it as their organ of special interest even though it accounts for about forty percent of the human body. Moreover, it counts for eighty-five percent of all chronic musculoskeletal pain, which is our most prevalent pain condition! One reason for this lack of interest might be that muscle pain is neither dangerous nor lethal—it only "kills" a lot of quality of life—and no pill or surgical method may cure it. So when it comes to muscle pain, we doctors cannot do what we love the most, namely saving lives and curing patients, as lasting pain relief lies, at the end of the day, in the hands of each patient. But the patients are dependent on the healthcare system to provide the necessary, individualized information to understand and know what to do! And here we doctors and physical therapists too often have failed them, due to lack of knowledge. As a physician, I learned very little about how to diagnose and treat muscle pain and muscle dysfunction during my medical studies. More surprisingly, I was no wiser in this area after finishing my specialization in *physical medicine and rehabilitation*. This was challenging to me, as musculoskeletal pain is the most frequent reason for adults to consult a medical doctor, and even more so in my specialty! It did not make it easier that muscle tissue causes a deep, diffuse pain that is difficult to localize, and also has a tendency to cause referred pain. Thus, you risk treating the wrong region if you are not acquainted with each muscle's referral patterns. Moreover, muscle pain cannot be revealed through conventional medical workups, blood testing, CT scans, or X-ray assessments. I felt helpless! So many of my patients suffered from severe pain while their medical assessments were completely normal, and I was not able to give them a satisfactory explanation or causative treatment. My feeble "I can't find anything wrong," or "this is probably just muscle pain," or "it is not dangerous, try to live as normally as possible and stay physically active," was just as unsatisfactory to my patients as it was to me.

In 1995, while working on my doctoral dissertation on fibromyalgia etiology and treatment, I attended the 3rd World Congress on Fibromyalgia and Myofascial Pain in San Antonio, Texas. Curious, I had signed up for a workshop on myofascial pain, a term previously unknown to me. There, the work of Dr. Janet Travell, M.D., and her way of clinically examining, diagnosing, and treating muscle pain was made known to me. I was thrilled! At last I had found what I had been sorely missing in my education so far! I also met myofascial pain therapist Nancy Shaw from Springfield, Virginia, who had been tutored by and worked closely together with Dr. Travell for thirteen years. Home in Norway again, I bought Drs. Travell and Simon's book: *Myofascial Pain and Dysfunction: The Trigger Point Manual.* Great reading! At last I had come one step further in providing my patients with a more accurate pain diagnosis, explanation, and advice on how to get rid of factors that could be perpetuating their pain.

In 2000, we designed a multidimensional, evidence-based rehabilitation program for patients with long-lasting, widespread pain and fibromyalgia at Jeløy Kurbad, in which we also wanted to include specific diagnostics and treatment of their muscle pain. There was no expertise for us to consult on this in Norway, but via the Internet, we were able to find Nancy Shaw and invite her over to teach our staff. Unbelievably, she closed down her practice for some weeks, brought along her coworkers, and came over! Seven times since 2001, she has visited in one- to two-week teaching and coaching sessions, always being a great source of inspiration and providing us with new, invaluable skills. She is a gifted teacher, a superb clinician—and wonderful person! She is so dedicated to helping patients and passing on her knowledge! Both our pain patients and staff have greatly benefited from the specific focus on myofascial pain diagnostics and treatment as part of our rehabilitation program. We provide our patients with knowledge and comprehension of their pain, and point out crucial perpetuating factors that have been preventing their recovery. Due to Nancy's help, we are able to give our patients a genuine chance for actively working on their way towards recovery! The challenge is now to spread this knowledge in the medical milieu! And here, this present book is a wonderful tool!

On various occasions, I have been fortunate to shadow Nancy dealing with patients at her own Myofascial Pain Treatment Center in Springfield, Virginia. She is a living extension of Dr. Janet Travell's knowledge, and the only therapist I know of that actually utilizes her full protocol. That is, Nancy not only releases the muscles that are causing the patients' pain, but has her main focus on *why* the pain is there. Searching for unique perpetuating factors, she has each of her patients bring photos of body postures from their daily life. By uncovering and changing factors that may cause and maintain their muscle dysfunction and pain, and demonstrating how to regain normal function, she gives her patients the possibility of permanent improvement and often, even total pain elimination! She asks, explains, demonstrates, motivates, and manually treats her patients as she educates and empowers them. And her aim is always the same: optimal and lasting pain relief!

Nancy Shaw's exceptional background and experience make her a leading expert in her field. Her years with Dr. Travell and her own lifelong clinical experience as a myofascial pain thera-pist and teacher in the field (teaching and educating healthcare providers on three continents) gives the firm foundation of this book. Her knowledge and skills in muscle function, perpetuat-ing factors, and stretching techniques are unique, and with this book she shares her work! The book has a very practical approach, with pictures and patient examples to make her points easy to grasp. She is communicating to her readers as she would have done had they been there per-sonally at her office. As this is a patient self-help book, the main focus is on body positions plus a section on stress. It thus addresses factors people may be able to change themselves without fur-ther professional help and does not intend to cover the complete area of perpetuating factors. After a short, general section on muscle pain and how to use the book, she presents her message in different sections based on various body positions that may be causing and perpetuating pain. Every section shows how different dysfunctional positions may affect and shorten specific mus-cles, together with the muscles' referred pain patterns. The reader is shown an alternative, more neutral body position to aim for, often with instructions on how to make the necessary change. Each section ends with a self-stretch program to reinforce a "muscle memory" that fits with the new postural habits being made. The sections are self-explanatory, making it possible to use the book as a manual, looking up specific areas of self-perceived pain only. Or you may read the book from beginning to end, and enjoy how Nancy describes the same principles in different ways, perceiving new aspects and nuances in the process. She writes in conversational language, understandable to all.

The present book is also unique from a medical point of view. To my knowledge, this is the first self-help book with a main focus on how to eliminate perpetuating factors for muscle pain, along with a tailored stretch-rehabilitation program. Furthermore, I have not found a single sci-entific myofascial pain treatment study that has included elimination of perpetuating factors as part of the intervention. This is strange, as Dr. Travell points out elimination of perpetuating fac-tors as the most crucial aspect when it comes to accomplishing long-lasting relief. My own experience from working with patients is in line with her statement. (I even got rid of my own recurring headaches and chronic shoulder pain by listening to Nancy!) But due to the lack of studies, there is so far no scientific evidence on the impact of perpetuating factors on chronic pain. It is however, not unlikely that the general tendency of neglecting perpetuating factors may have a say in our great number of chronic pain sufferers! From Dr. Travell's experience, patients may get rid of seventy-five percent of their pain solely by eliminating their perpetuating factors and by performing stretching exercises. But they need to know *how*, and that is what this patient self-help book is all about! This is what also makes *Simple Changes To End Chronic Pain* such a valuable asset for everyone, including physicians, physical therapists, and other healthcare workers. It presents practical information on reasons for muscle pain, what to look for, and how to instruct patients, provided that a thorough medical workup has ruled out all other possible causes for their pain. The latter is a most crucial step that cannot be overlooked! Both patients and healthcare providers need to be aware of the possibility of missing potentially dangerous and treatable underlying disease by skipping the medical workup and prematurely assuming the pain to be of muscular origin alone.

In conclusion, this unique patient self-help book offers ordinary people and the medical milieu a key to understanding and treating diffuse musculoskeletal pain, where no obvious etiology has been found. It meets a long-existing gap in common medical knowledge and may even inspire scientists to perform the studies needed to give this field an evidence-based foundation. I thus recommend *Simple Changes To End Chronic Pain* to all who want to get rid of muscle pain and stiffness, chronic pain sufferers and healthcare providers alike!

One last point: if you want to get the most from this book, do exactly as Nancy advices! By under- or overdoing, you risk losing valuable improvement possibilities.

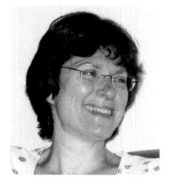

Ski, June 2013
Sigrid Hørven Wigers, MD, PhD, CMTPT
Consultant and Rehabilitation Manager
Jeløy Kurbad, Moss, Norway

Welcome

These days, many people spend much of their day sitting, standing, or sleeping. Do those things correctly the majority of the time, and your body will allow for those few times of doing something differently.

I wrote this book to share valuable information with you who are living with daily aches and pains, muscle stiffness, uneasiness, and weakness that affect your life in various ways. The way you use your body can cause pain, and I want to show you how simple changes can eliminate that pain. I want to share lessons I have learned personally from instances in my own life, as well as lessons I learned from years with my mentor, Janet G. Travell, M.D., White House physician to President John F. Kennedy. Dr. Travell won a Lifetime Achievement Award from the American Academy of Pain Management for pioneering the medical field of myofascial pain and dysfunction. I've spent over thirty years applying the truths she presented, truths about *muscles and how they function* that confirm the power you can have over chronic pain. There is nothing I know of that works better. I was thrilled to receive the following correspondence from Dr. Travell in 1993:

> *"Nancy, I want you to know that I highly regard your expertise in the control of myofascial pain and dysfunction with improvement in the quality of life of your patients, and how impressed I am by your successful efforts to bring myotherapy into the mainstream of medicine."*

The book in your hands will allow you to experience those same truths that I learned from Dr. Travell. Through pictures and examples, you will probably recognize yourself in one way or another. It is knowledge and then discipline, not desire, which will take you to a place of pain-free living. My goal is for you to become aware of what pain you may have and to tune into what you're doing that may be causing it. I will show you how to make simple changes, changes that can end your chronic pain. It will be a choice, a choice I hope you will make.

I look at chronic pain differently than many: I don't think that most chronic pain is due to something *wrong* with the body. I believe pain is the downside of your muscles' developing various degrees of tightness that results in their being out of balance when you use them. I believe that the vast majority of chronic pain involves muscles that have learned to function incorrectly. In cases where muscle dysfunction causes chronic pain, pain is not something that needs to be *managed or adjusted to.* Rather, it calls for identifying what muscle imbalances have occurred and figuring out what led to those imbalances. Then you can make necessary changes to the way you use your muscles and teach them to work in a coordinated, balanced pattern.

Where does this muscle tightness come from? You may know people who have experienced serious accidents, falls, surgeries, injuries, and illnesses that left a lot of pain hanging around, becoming chronic. It's clear where that pain comes from. On the other hand, you may know others who do not know where their pain comes from, and who wonder why they have it. You may be one of them. Did you know that just normal daily use of muscles can create tension in them that can eventually result in pain? While it does matter where chronic pain comes from, when it becomes chronic, it generally involves muscles that have learned to function incorrectly, and that should be the focus of treatment. If that is the case, it means you can be in control, whether the pain results from any number of causes, or from an unknown source: you can learn what muscles are not functioning correctly or are out of balance, and can make changes that will help diminish or eliminate that imbalance and, therefore, the pain.

Why do I feel so certain about this? Let me share an event that showcased the muscle-function-and-dysfunction approach and proved to me that there are answers even when something catastrophic has occurred.

In 2005, I was involved in a most unexpected accident, one that moved me from being a therapist to being a patient. I had become an avid cyclist and had done some great biking that summer. It was October when I left for a long weekend of biking on Cape Cod, off season and perfect for a picturesque adventure. On a beautiful sunny day I put on my helmet and yellow shirt, and set out for a ride. I was only fifteen or twenty minutes into that first day of riding when I was struck from behind by a car traveling about forty miles per hour. I didn't see it coming. What I remember is my back exploding in pain on impact. The next thing I knew, I lay on my side, half on and half off the road, curled up and struggling to breathe. I couldn't get air into my lungs. The pain was excruciating, and I remember saying "my back is broken, I can't breathe." I knew I was alive, but I also knew it was bad.

At the hospital, I was told I had multiple anterior compression back fractures and a burst fracture at the mid-point of my thoracic spine. I also had several rib fractures, two fractures in my ankle, muscle and tendon damage in my leg and ankle, shattered bones in my thumb, fluid in my lung, and lots of bruises and scrapes.

No one quite knew what the recovery would be, but thank God, I was alive. That was the miracle for me. I was alive, and I could still think and feel. At the time, though, what I was also feeling was a lot of pain.

I was aware that rehabilitation would be slow and difficult. Much of my spine would be permanently rounded or bent forward (kyphosis), with my neck following in a forward position. This meant that my *muscles,* rather than my spine, would need to do extra work to hold me upright. That was my ultimate goal, to be as upright as possible, and to be *functional:* to be able to work, play, travel, and enjoy life once again, as I had before.

I talked with my physicians, and they agreed to allow me to do my own rehabilitation therapy, giving me sound medical advice along the way. I used the principles of the *muscle function and dysfunction protocol* I present in this book: muscle dysfunction retraining through simple postural changes and stretching.

I knew the accident would change my life, but I didn't want it to dictate my future—and it didn't. Today I am thoroughly enjoying a full and active life, including biking, cross-country skiing, teaching other therapists, and running a busy practice treating myofascial chronic pain.

When I set out on that bike ride, I had no idea that my life would soon be headed in a different direction. But I am grateful that out of a terrible accident, I've become empowered to help others even more fully than I previously did in my pain clinic. I have a deep understanding of the challenges facing patients who have pain resulting from trauma, surgery, or even from leaning over all day at a job. And I am committed, through this book, to sharing my expertise and tips to drastically reduce or eliminate those frustrating aches, pains, and chronic movement limitations you may suffer needlessly.

You may already know what causes some of the muscle imbalances that create or affect your pain, or you may be in the dark. More importantly, you may be ready to make the changes I suggest in the book that are necessary to decrease or eliminate that pain. For those who are not ready, I hope you will read this book and come to the time when you will learn and embrace the changes and enjoy a new-found freedom. I want to show you that the postural and movement changes needed are simple ones that can give you back the pain-free life you used to enjoy. But like all changes, they may feel awkward at first. With patience and practice, they'll soon become natural.

So now it is your turn. It is your turn to begin your journey to wellness. Just turn the page. We can make this book an adventure, a journey we take together. It is my sincerest wish that you will be as excited as I am about the new direction of your life, your life without chronic pain. May you once again enjoy the simple pleasures of life!

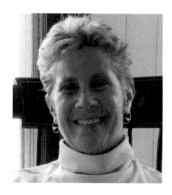

August 2013
Nancy Lee Shaw, M.S., M.A., MTPT
Director
Myofascial Pain Treatment Center
Springfield, Virginia

Chapter 1.
The "Whys" of Chronic Pain

Chronic pain is something you hear about a great deal. People ask, "Why do so many people hurt nowadays, with aches and pains or more serious, chronic, long-lasting pain?" It is true that a lot of people have chronic pain, despite having gone to some kind of therapy, and having taken who knows how many medications. Medically, there seems to be a general lack of consensus on treatment for many types of pain. It is no wonder people are confused about what really works. I frequently hear, "I just don't get it. With all the advances in modern medicine, why is chronic pain still around?"

Of course, there are people with cancer or neurological and other conditions that deal with daily pain as a part of their situation. Pain may also be experienced by people with injuries or permanent structural problems. But what about those without such specific conditions who still experience chronic pain, even on a daily basis?

"I've had my back evaluated by everyone, with every kind of treatment attempted that you can think of."

"My shoulder and arm have been in a sling, I've quit lifting anything heavy, I've gone to the gym to strengthen my shoulder, I've even had arthroscopy, and I still can't lift my arm very high without a lot of pain."

"My knees hurt all the time, even after injections, braces, and strengthening exercises."

These comments or some variation of them, made by patients when they come to my clinic for treatment, are a good indication of the ongoing pain problem. So what are we missing?

In the August—September 2012 issue of the *AARP Bulletin*, it was noted that 100 million people in the United States live with chronic pain, at a cost of $635 billion a year. They live with the aches and pains and "tightness" that most people think are "normal," a fact of life, a part of "getting older." Doesn't everyone have some arthritis, achy knees and shoulders, backaches, the occasional headache? Doesn't life catch up with us and leave us with things like carpal tunnel syndrome, rotator cuff strains, plantar fasciitis, bulging discs, tennis elbow, and frozen shoulders? Don't most people wake up stiff and sore, needing a hot shower and a bit of moving around to loosen up? Isn't that "just life"? Because we believe this, we may just keep on doing the same things over and over, adapting as best we can, and hoping we might get different results: less pain. Unfortunately, that doesn't usually happen!

The big question is: why?

Why is it so difficult to think of life without chronic pain? Is it because so many people, often including you, experience chronic pain? If you believed life could exist without chronic pain, wouldn't it make sense to be willing to make simple changes in how you use your body and to teach your muscles how to function correctly? Chronic pain has been labeled a complex problem—addressed by a variety of medications, extensive therapy and body work, and shared among support groups—all without resolution. You may try to learn to live with chronic pain, change your lifestyle, reduce your activities, and even change professions, *but* you still have chronic pain.

As chronic aches and pains become more frequent and more intense over time, they need to be evaluated differently than in the past. Your body is made up of many muscles that are all meant to function in balance with each other. If just one muscle gets out of balance, it will directly or indirectly affect the others. Muscles, working in groups, need to maintain their ability to stretch freely and still to contract in strength to avoid overload and vulnerability to pain that can become chronic. Treatment is often aimed at eliminating the pain *symptoms* at the site of the pain, but without lasting resolution of the pain that people experience. Too often, relief is only temporary.

It is time to look beyond the symptoms of chronic pain and to focus on the cause, on *why* the knee, shoulder, or back hurts; and *where* the pain is coming from. Doctors look for structural or physical reasons for pain. When nothing is found on the X-rays, MRIs, or other tests and evaluations, the tendency is to treat symptoms. After all, the patient simply wants the pain gone.

But what if the answer is simple, but elusive? What if a majority of chronic pain is really related to muscles: how muscles function, why they begin to function improperly, and how you accommodate improper function in ways that perpetuate the problem?

The noted Chief White House Physician, Janet G. Travell, M.D., put forth this dysfunctional muscle approach fifty years ago, yet never saw its validity accepted. Why? Perhaps because physicians focus on structural issues or muscle damage rather than muscular dysfunction. That is what they are trained to do, and do well. It would make sense, then, that if pain involves muscular dysfunction, the pain would not show up as the result of any definite structural problem or muscle damage on any examination or test performed. When the medical workup looks normal, only the symptoms are addressed. However, treating symptoms may make you feel better for a short time, but the cause of the chronic pain still must be determined and eliminated for you to stay pain free.

Interestingly, no field of medicine directly claims *muscle function and dysfunction* as a specialty. As noted, doctors are not trained to deal with function, per se; they are trained to address structural problems and injury or damage to the body. When the structure shows no reason for pain, someone trained specifically in function and not only in symptom relief needs to become involved in evaluation and treatment.

Today's approach to chronic pain relief has not led to consistent results of pain elimination, nor even successful pain management. If it had, we would not have near-epidemic levels of chronic pain in this country, with almost a third of the population of the United States reporting that their lives have been affected. A different approach may be most helpful!

A New Approach: Overview

Chronic pain usually involves *muscles and their function* that form a pattern when performing tasks. There are many aspects to what you do with your muscles, and why you do these things. Chronic pain is complex because by the time it becomes chronic, it has invaded many aspects of the person's life: physical, mental, emotional, psychological, financial, occupational, social, and recreational. Each category mentioned can be further broken down into subcategories. Whew! To gather all the pieces of the pain puzzle, it is important to investigate all the components of your life to elicit the clues to pain resolution. How do you begin to unravel the puzzle of your chronic pain?

Muscles

Let's take a new look at *muscle function and dysfunction.* Muscles contract and release as we go through our daily activities, whether driving, reading, working at a desk, or running for the bus. If they contract more than they release, tension builds and you feel tight. Do you *listen* to your muscles or body at that time? Not really—after all, doesn't everyone experience tight muscles? Yes, but because muscles are capable of developing a "memory," they are capable of developing habits of functioning long or short; that is, properly or improperly. If muscles are short (that is, tight), they function improperly. The muscles thus become weaker because they are shorter than normal, and therefore lose muscle capacity to do the work asked of them. They also fatigue easily, because they are trying to do normal tasks with less muscle ability available. It takes a lot more energy to accomplish even routine tasks with shortened muscles, and pain eventually settles in. Exercising to strengthen the muscles at this point will only increase the tightness and may increase the pain.

Let's look even further into the muscle aspect of pain. You probably have heard of *myofascial* treatment. *Myo* = muscle, and *fascia* = connective tissue, which runs throughout the body to hold everything together. Connective tissue can get bound up when you have tight muscles. Myofascial treatment, therefore, simply means *any* treatment aimed at the muscles and connective tissue. These treatments, however, often give only temporary relief, because the focus of treatment is where the patient feels the pain, at the *pain site.* This approach is an attempt to relax the muscles, as well as release any connective tissue binding. But this alone does not eliminate the pain for a prolonged period. The pain often returns. Let's look even deeper.

You may have heard of *trigger points.* A trigger point is a hyper-irritable spot located in a taut band of a muscle. The spot is painful when pressure is applied to that specific point in the muscle. In addition, most trigger points have a *referred pain pattern,* which means the pain can be felt somewhere other than where you find the trigger point. Referred pain may be felt in a joint or in a muscle some distance away from 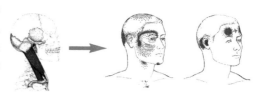 the trigger point. Focusing on the pain pattern can lead us to the *origin* of the pain. Treating the

Muscle causing pai   **Pain site**

muscle that is short and is the underlying cause of the pain, rather than the site where you feel the pain, is the key to permanent relief.

The location of trigger points and their corresponding referred pain sites are scientifically documented in the medical texts *Myofascial Pain and Dysfunction: The Trigger Point Manual, Vols. 1 and 2,* authored by Janet G. Travell, M.D., and David G. Simons, M.D. These documented pain patterns are available to help locate the *source* of your pain: which muscle is short and is referring pain.

You must understand the pain resulting from muscle tightness and the elicited referral patterns as you seek to eliminate your chronic pain. Some of the referral patterns will not seem logical, nor will they be familiar to you. That is why the work of documenting these patterns is such a treasure. This simple approach addresses the "why" of pain: what is causing your pain to continue and become chronic. Fifty-odd years later, Dr. Travell's approach is still the proven roadmap to resolving chronic pain. Below are interesting tidbits gleaned from her work, regarding muscles that frequently cause muscle pain and where that pain is experienced:

- Chronic *back pain* often results from repeated shortening of two muscles, the rectus abdominus and iliopsoas, both muscles attaching in the *front* of the body—yes, back pain from muscles in the front. These two muscles help perform such movements as bending forward or lifting the leg and bringing it toward the chest. These movements shorten the muscles in the front but exhibit a back pain pattern. It is critical, then, to evaluate how you sleep, sit to read and watch television, and sit at the computer and in the car. Evaluating these postures helps to determine if you are slouching, drawing your knees up, rounding the back, or bending forward in a way that shortens these muscles and results in back pain.

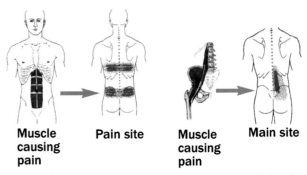

Muscle causing pain   Pain site   Muscle causing pain   Main site

- *Headaches* are commonly caused by strained or shortened neck and upper back muscles that result from sleeping in a faulty posture, sitting slouched in a recliner or on a soft sofa with the shoulders and head pushed forward, or watching television or reading while lying down.

Muscle causing pain   Pain site

- *Plantar fasciitis*, a painful inflammation on the bottom of the foot, is often a result of improper shoes (e.g., stiff or inflexible) and faulty gait or walking movements.

- *Frozen shoulder* necessitates evaluating sleep position, overload of the muscles when performing activities such as gardening, yard work, painting, cleaning the car, doing housework, or carrying purses or backpacks on one shoulder.

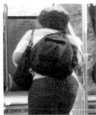

What do these scenarios have in common? Each involves improper postures or repeated and frequent misuse of muscles, accommodating tightness and teaching the muscles an improper way of functioning. Even without totally understanding the scientific physiology behind these pain patterns, you can be certain that trigger points are part of your pain. So, is treating trigger points the answer to getting rid of chronic pain? Yes—and no. Let's look at other issues before answering that question.

Perpetuating Factors

Treating the *source* of pain, the muscle that is tight, involves another important aspect: *perpetuating factors. Identifying perpetuating factors holds the key to permanent muscle pain elimination.* Perpetuating factors are the most commonly overlooked issues in treatment but may be easier to understand than the *source* of pain. So, what are they? The easiest way to explain perpetuating factors is to say that they are what you do when you hurt, to try to make yourself more comfortable. For example, you change how you sit: your chair may be too big for you or your sofa too soft, inviting you to slouch or sit with a leg tucked under you. Your computer is set off to the side on your desk, and the desktop is too low to allow you to pull up close, so you start lean forward and twist in your chair to see the monitor. The back of the desk chair slants backward, so you lean forward and prop yourself with chin in hand. You shoes have stiff soles that don't bend, so you walk flat-footed, lifting your hip to allow your leg to swing forward.

These examples of *adaptations* to your surroundings and *accommodations* to your situation set in motion how you will sleep at night. You will sleep in postures that reflect the way you sat and walked. You will sleep curled, mimicking slouching and leaning forward at your desk. Your shoe *accommodation* may include buying different shoes, but you also *adapt* to the situation as you switch from running to biking and from walking to swimming. The accommodations and adaptations are never ending. You will automatically do what you need to do with work or home situations, and then change what you need to in order to be as comfortable as possible. *These adaptations and accommodations become perpetuating factors.* Now it is important to see what the consequences of these accommodations and adaptations are.

Accommodations and Adaptations. More about accommodations. First, as mentioned previously, you have to recognize that muscle tightness occurs from normal use, all the things you do every day. All the ways in which you use your muscles without relaxing them are factors that result in the muscles' becoming and staying tight. Tight muscles are not comfortable, so you begin the accommodations and adjustments that can add more tension to your muscles. *What you have done to be comfortable is now what has taught the muscles to stay short:* the postures you use for sleeping, watching television, reading, working on the computer, driving your car, working on your hobbies, and participating in leisure activities. These factors, and others, can be involved in *why* you experience chronic pain on a regular basis!

Accommodations and adaptations feel good. Remember, back pain can be referred pain from muscles in the front of the body. Of course, a *bending forward posture* (bending over the sink to brush your teeth) then feels good, because the muscles in the front of the body are already short from postures such as your sitting *slouched* (sitting with the body rounded over your desk). You

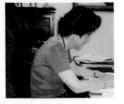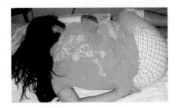

shorten the same muscles whether you are sitting slouched or bending forward, so both postures become equally comfortable. But that doesn't mean the adaptations are good for you. Muscles *learn* patterns of function. Slouching or bending forward repeatedly during the day helps the muscle make a *habit* of that posture. Then, if you choose to sleep in a curled posture, you will simply continue to teach the muscles to function in that habitual short pattern.

The curled posture will feel normal because you have already trained the muscles to be short by slouching and bending forward during the day. But these postures all shorten the same muscles in the lower abdomen and the hip, no matter which you choose. The result is the same: the muscles *learn* to be shorter and shorter, reinforced by your accommodating postures. Repeatedly using the muscles in a shortened position will establish a *muscle memory* of working short. Spinal changes, as seen here, and pain will result when the abdominal and hip

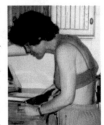

muscles shorten to the point that they start eliciting referred pain to the back. I will keep reminding you that back pain is referred from muscles in the front of the body. Really grasping that fact will help eliminate one of the most universal chronic pain problems; that is, low-back pain, experienced in most countries.

Until the muscles relearn to function in a longer position, movement will be restricted and painful when you try to use shortened muscles to stand up straight, as when getting out of bed or rising from a sitting posture. Short muscles can even cause back pain when you stand longer than usual, because they are not used to being held in the unfamiliar, longer position. Muscles will continue to function in their short position until you teach them to elongate. This is done by stretching on a regular basis.

Hands-on treatment alone for this back pain cannot eliminate the pain you may feel when you get out of bed in the morning. The pain is now the result of daytime slouching and the curled sleeping posture that reinforced the shortness of the muscles that are referring pain to your back. Instead of hands-on treatment, you have to change accommodating postures to a more neu-

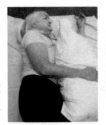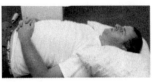

tral, elongated posture: the body straight, the head in line with the body, and the legs only slightly bent when sleeping. Then the muscles will *learn* to be long again, and will stay long throughout the day and during the night. It is these changes—new sleeping, sitting, and standing postures, reinforced by muscle retraining with specific stretches—that can eliminate your back pain.

Here's another example of change that brings positive results. If you play a sport or regularly participate in an activity—if you play golf, for example—you may think your clubs are fine and feel as though you have a decent swing. But your score isn't the best. So how do you improve? You take lessons from a professional and discover your clubs are too long, and your swing, well, let's just say it needs help! You learn what changes you need to make. You get the right equipment and then practice and practice, until you establish a new *muscle memory* for your swing and watch your score improve. You changed the perpetuating factors that were keeping your swing inadequate, and practiced to eliminate the problem.

Adaptations and accommodations that you may not even be aware of can be perpetuating factors that can have you stuck in chronic pain. To help discover your perpetuating factors, have someone take photographs of you in your sleeping postures, watching television, reading, sitting at the computer and in the car, carrying bags, working at your job or at home, and anything else you do frequently, such as hobbies or activities. This will give you a snapshot of what accommodations or adaptations you are making to try to be comfortable. Once you identify the changes necessary to obtain neutral and relaxed body posturing shown throughout this book, practice these changes. You will notice your pain beginning to go away.

> **Change is easy: it's thinking about change that's hard.**
> —Dr. Eric Plasker, *The 100 Year Lifestyle*

Dr. Travell often said that identifying perpetuating factors like accommodations was the most critical aspect of her treatment protocol, contributing at least seventy-five percent to the elimination or prevention of chronic muscle pain. In the medical text, regarding the chapter on *perpetuating factors*, she stated: *"This is the most important single chapter in this manual: it concerns the most neglected part of the management of myofascial pain syndrome* [chronic muscle pain]." Eliminating perpetuating factors is mandatory for reversing chronic pain on a permanent basis.

Why then, if perpetuating factors can be identified and reduced or eliminated, do so many people suffer from chronic pain unnecessarily? Why is pain the norm? Why is it such an accepted part of life? There are a number of reasons why this is so. Remember that pain affects your entire being, not just where you hurt. It infiltrates every part of you. It is so omnipresent that people accept pain as something that is just a part of life.

Let's take a look at some of the common *categories of perpetuating factors* invading every part of your life that can prevent you from eliminating your pain. I have put this in a pie chart with "Pain" in the middle.

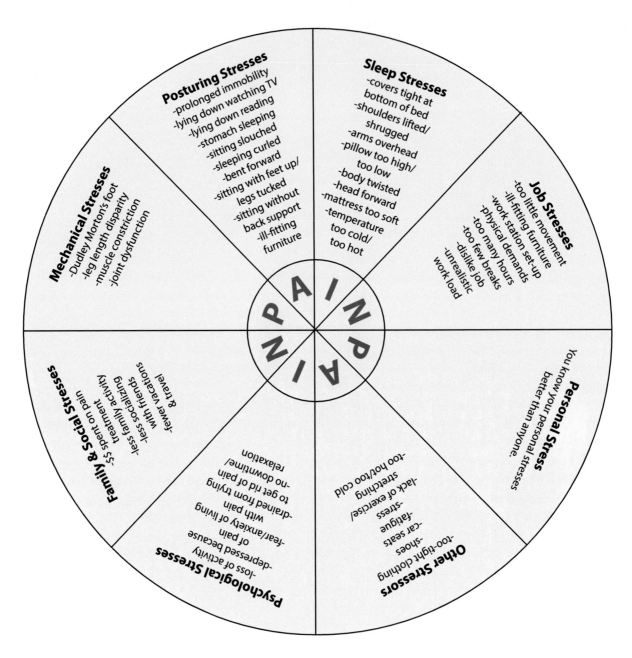

No matter how you look at it, it's pain!

Looking at this diagram, patients often say, "But if you'll just fix my pain, everything else will be okay."

What you have to understand is that pain is in the *middle* of the pie. All these categories of perpetuating factors contain pieces of your pain. If you fix only one or two categories, you fix only part of the pain. It is so important that we look together at *all* of the categories to identify the changes you need to make to eliminate your pain.

Others might say, "My aches and pains are just a part of everyday living, and a part of growing old. Nothing I can do about it."

"It's true," I tell them, "that what you do contributes to your aches and pains, but it's really what you don't do that is the real culprit behind your pain. You don't stretch!" Using your muscles during the day results in their holding a lot of tension. They should relax, returning to a neutral position when you are not using them. The problem is that as you use your muscles and then relax, the muscles normally retain a little bit of the tension. If you were simply to stretch the muscles occasionally, they could return to a longer, more neutral position. If you continue to contract the muscles without intentionally stretching, however, the muscles will learn to stay in a shortened position. They'll begin to feel *normal* in this shortened state.

Try this experiment:

1. Start with a full open hand position.

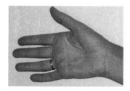

2. Make a fist (go ahead and try it) and hold it a few seconds.

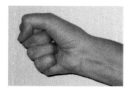

3. Release it by letting go of the fist.

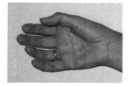

Notice that your fingers do not automatically return to their original, fully open starting position. They stop short of their full extension.

4. Start the next contraction from that slightly shortened position, hold it a few seconds, and then relax.

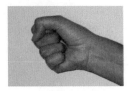

5. The hand will retain more tension, more tightness, returning to an even tighter, shorter position.

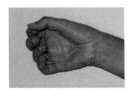

Without some intervention, the process will repeat itself, gradually shortening the muscles' range of motion more and more. This happens to muscles everywhere in the body, making them shorter and shorter, preventing them from returning to a full open resting position.

Without adequate stretching to re-lengthen the muscles, tightness and shortness continue to increase. Once the muscles are shortened (tight), they are no longer free to be used to full capability. You continue using the muscles until one more movement produces *pain*, even severe pain. You think the pain happened all of a sudden. Instead, it resulted from the gradual buildup of tightness in the muscle, to the point that one more bit of tension was too much, and pain resulted. Because the last movement resulted in pain, it appears as if it is *suddenly* difficult and painful to stand straight, turn your head as far as you should, or climb the steps as fast as you did before. This pain, however, is the result of the accumulation of shortness or tension in the muscles over days, weeks, months, or even years. You have used the muscles and done little to move them back to their original, more extended, neutral position, which would give them full use potential. You have not stretched!

Remember, along with producing pain, shortened muscles are *weak* and *fatigue* more easily, as they try to perform from a slightly contracted position. This type of muscle weakness does not indicate the need for strength work. It is a "false weakness." The muscles are not strong because they are too tight. This tightness, or shortness, indicates a need to stretch your muscles to regain their full strength, so they may be used again from their full neutral and open position.

Muscles have *memory*. They do whatever you teach them. Do enough of the same thing with a muscle, and that posture or movement becomes the *muscle habit*. If you don't stretch muscles frequently, they get too short and develop a memory of functioning short, or tight. The muscle develops *muscle memory* from repetition of all your automatic movements: walking, standing, sitting, bending, reaching, climbing stairs, playing sports, and doing everything else you do. All muscles function according to the habits you have taught them. If those habits promote shortened muscles, the muscles become vulnerable to pain. Let me explain it with the following diagram:

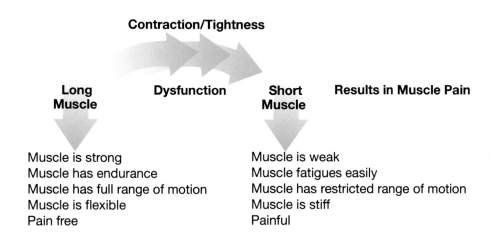

Contraction/Tightness

| **Long Muscle** | **Dysfunction** | **Short Muscle** | **Results in Muscle Pain** |

Muscle is strong
Muscle has endurance
Muscle has full range of motion
Muscle is flexible
Pain free

Muscle is weak
Muscle fatigues easily
Muscle has restricted range of motion
Muscle is stiff
Painful

As the muscle shortens, aches and pains begin to invade your daily life. You handle these aches and pains by changing your lifestyle. But life shouldn't be about doing less and less, and giving up what you like to do. It should be about finding the source of the problem, changing what needs to be changed, and returning to a full and pain-free life.

As you use muscles and tightness builds in an area—say, around a knee—you start a cascade involving other muscles as they try to help or protect the tight muscles. Let's say you begin to put more weight on the other leg, maybe even limping a little. Well, you can see where this is going. You begin to feel tightness and pain in the opposite hip and leg as well because of the overload. Your feet begin to get sore, so you change the way you walk. You have accommodated for the knee pain and adjusted how you use your body, trying to make it through the day.

This chain of changes may soon result in strain and stresses throughout your body. You slouch a bit when you are sitting, lean against something when you are standing, change shoes before a walk, grab a different pillow when you go to bed, and end up sleeping in any position that is comfortable. You try anything to feel good again, even though you have a feeling it may not be the best posture. You get really desperate because things are spiraling out of control. Everything you try seems to make the pain worse.

The descending spiral of tightness, and the stress it causes in the muscles, eventually turns into the aches and pains that sap your energy. Many people have several spirals going at the same time. As a consequence, the muscles have you making compromises, such as beginning to eliminate certain movements and stopping participation in favorite activities, which leave you living a life different from the one you envisioned.

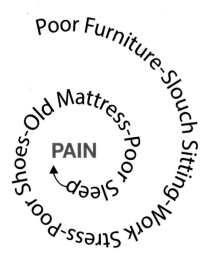

Patients tell me they quit doing many of the things they used to do, thinking that if they just rest and wait it out, the pain will eventually go away. That resting time may help decrease the pain simply because you are not using the involved muscles, but it doesn't take long for the pain to return. Why? You would think that not doing the painful movements or activities would help a lot. *Note that resting does not work.* When muscles have "learned" bad habits, and you do nothing but rest them, the muscles have the same pain-producing habits as before. As soon as you begin your activities again, the muscles function in those same, incorrect, learned patterns. You did not change anything by not using the muscles, so you really couldn't expect them to know any better. They continue to do what they used to do that caused pain. Same habits, same pain!

Ending chronic pain is a process that has the same starting point for everyone. You first *identify* the *postures* you use frequently, as they are presented in this book. Next, you *identify* the short *muscles* and the *referred pain patterns* that are indicated in the postural sections on sleeping, sitting, and standing. Next, you note the *perpetuating factors*, the *accommodations* (things like furniture, shoes, or beds) you are using that may be causing your muscles to shorten or to stay tight. This tightness, in turn, may cause you to use some odd postures. The odd postures are *adaptations*, or changed positions that you have taken to be as comfortable as possible. Postures that allow muscles to be more relaxed and in a neutral, elongated position are essential to eliminating your pain. Stretching frequently throughout the day helps teach the muscles to function in correct ways and helps maintain this longer, more neutral muscle position.

The next questions a patient might ask are, "I can certainly change what I do if you can help me figure out the problem. Is that all I have to do? How long will it take to feel good again?"

How long it takes to improve and become pain free depends on the time it takes to accomplish three things. First, it is necessary to *identify* all the perpetuating factors, the accommodations and adaptations you are consistently using. Second, you must *eliminate* these perpetuating factors that are roadblocks to good muscle function and "feeling good." Remember, this book will help you identify specific changes you need to make and give suggestions so you can succeed in *making* them. The final, critical step is to begin *lengthening,* or *stretching,* your muscles, retraining them to work at their full capacity.

As you correct your accommodating sleeping, sitting, and standing postures, you will automatically begin to lengthen the muscles. Stretching frequently makes the shift to elongated working muscles happen more quickly and prevents the muscles from returning to old shortened habits. Stretches are presented with each section to help you retrain your muscles, establishing good muscle function. The time it takes for you to accomplish these three steps will determine how soon your pain can be eliminated.

Stretch. Let me talk for a minute about stretching. *Stretching must become a part of your daily activities, just like eating and sleeping. Regular moments of stretching throughout the day are required for muscles to maintain a balanced capability. If you neglect regular muscle lengthening just because the pain is gone, the muscles will simply begin their old way of working, accumulating tightness, bit by bit, that will start the spiral into chronic pain all over again.*

Some patients respond, "Oh, that's no problem. I stretch every morning and when I work out. Besides, I heard it's good to use those rubber-type bands for stretching. I tried that, but it hasn't made much difference in my pain. In fact, it may have made it a little worse."

Let me explain the difference between the kind of stretching you may be used to doing, and the concept of stretching discussed and used in this book. It may be a new and entirely different activity for you. It is not about working out stiff muscles in the morning nor about a workout warm-up. Remember, we are doing muscle retraining, changing *muscle memory*, for the purpose of gaining full use of muscles, free from tightness or shortness in a resting position. Using elastic exercise bands for stretching can add resistance and increase tightness, when your goal is muscle relaxation and elongation. Resistance works against creating new *muscle memory*. The bands work fine for muscle strengthening, but not for the kind of stretching that eliminates shortness in the muscle.

The stretching you will learn in this book is all about frequency and new *muscle habits*. Do anything enough times, and it becomes a learned pattern, a habit. These stretches involve two repetitions and will only take a couple of minutes of your time.

The *basic principles* of the stretch program are simple, governed by *The Rule of Two:*

2-Repetitions: Perform only two repetitions of each stretch you are given.

2-Breaths: Hold the stretch and take two slow, deep breaths. This lets the brain and the body know everything is okay, and the muscles begin to release their tightness as you do the stretch.

2-Sides: Stretch both sides of the body, not just the painful side, to restore balance in the body. Stretch each side separately, as one side may be tighter than the other.

2-Hours: Repeat the stretches every two hours. Remember, it is the frequency that teaches new function.

Here are some basic *focus points* for performing a stretch correctly:

- This is a *feel-good* stretch, not a *see-how-far-you-can-push* stretch.
- Don't rush the stretch; feel the muscle's response to the stretch movement.
- Feel a slight stretch, avoiding a hard pull on the muscle.
- Hold the stretch gently. It should feel good.
- Hold the stretch steady, avoiding bouncing.

Try to keep the body as loose and relaxed as possible as you stretch. Feeling that looseness at first may be difficult, but it will come as the muscles are freed from tightness. Just keep breathing deeply for your two breaths.

This book will give you the stretches to do. They are specific to the changes you are making as you eliminate the accommodations and adaptations you have been using to control your pain.

The stretches require no specific equipment or facility. They are designed so you can do them easily whether you are at work, at home, or out and about.

"Is it really as easy as it sounds?" patients ask.

It is—and the really neat thing is that by making the changes and stretching, *you* are now in control of your pain. *You* can choose to make the changes or not. You can choose to stretch or not. The decision to do these three things—identify the short muscles, eliminate the accommodations, and stretch to retrain the muscles—puts *you* in the driver's seat.

This book will give you the tools for identifying, changing, and retraining problem muscles. Your biggest challenge will be your willingness to change. Thinking about change is not enough. Part-time changes and stretches are not enough. Life can be better; you get to choose. Choose and then act. It is an exciting adventure, which I look forward to sharing with you.

Notes

How This Book Works!

Start with Pictures

Have someone take the following photographs of you: Sleep postures, sitting watching television, reading, sitting at the computer, eating, in your car, and in any hobbies or activities.

Identify your posture in the book!

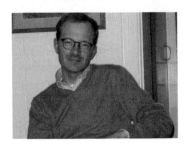 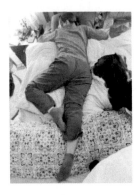 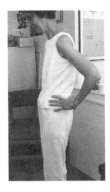

See what muscles you tighten in that posture!

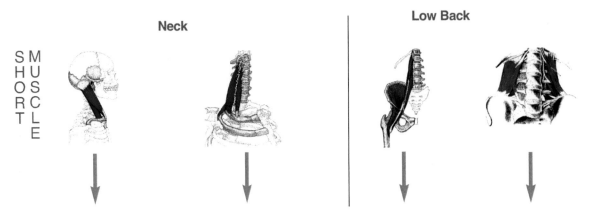

Notice the pain these tight muscles elicit!

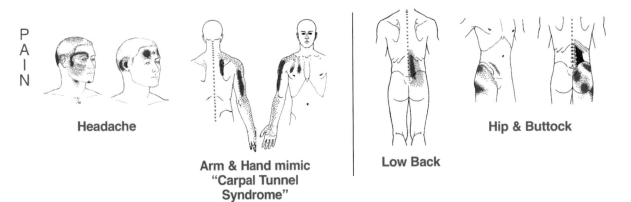

Win Pain-free Living
by Changing Postures

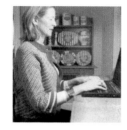 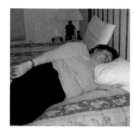 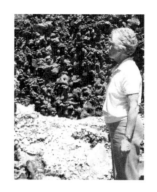

and stretching, stretching, stretching!

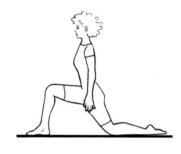 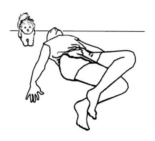 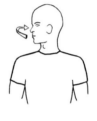

Simple, but effective!

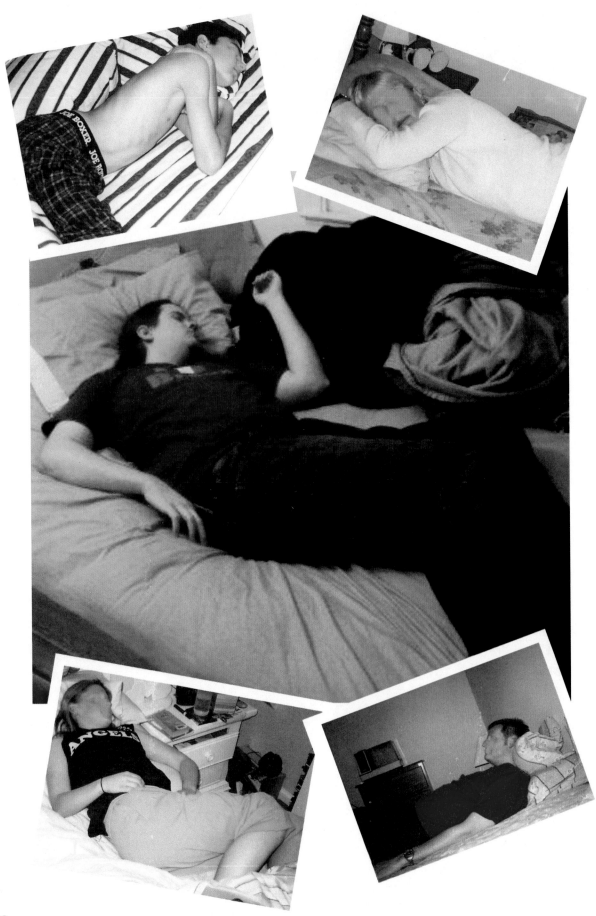

Chapter 2.
Sleep: Your Pain Story Told in Pictures

*T*he following scenarios are drawn from three patient consultations. You will begin to see a pattern in the approach used to identify perpetuating factors and accommodations involved in causing pain that can become chronic.

John. John called the clinic at the suggestion of a friend, hoping to get rid of the headaches that had plagued him for months. "The headaches usually start at night, and by morning can be so severe it can take an hour or more for them to ease enough that I can go to work. They don't always last all day, but always seem to come back during the night. I have tried several treatments, but nothing lasts more than a day or two. My friend said you helped him, so I thought I would give you a try."

I assured John we would take a different approach than he had tried before. To get started, I asked John to bring in photographs of his sleep postures, as well as of him in the evening on the sofa or in a recliner. Taking a look at the way he positions his muscles will help understand what may be contributing to his headaches. Reviewing the pictures will help John become more aware of postures that may teach muscles to function incorrectly, producing pain.

"You mean you want to see my X-rays and MRI films?" John asked.

"No," I said, "I want someone at home to take pictures of all the positions in which you sleep, doze off in the evening, or catch a quick nap. You don't have to be asleep; the photos just need to show the furniture and postures that you use. I need to see what you're doing with your muscles that might be the cause of your headaches."

John brought the pictures to his first appointment, and, well, the pictures *did* tell the story: John *sleeps "flat-out" on his stomach.*

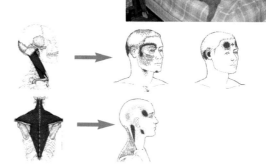

"John," I said, "with your head turned to the side all night, you're shortening the neck and upper-back muscles. When you hold these muscles so short (tight), they can produce headaches. You will need to break that habit of stomach sleeping in order to eliminate the muscle strain that is causing your headaches."

"What if I can't do it and just keep rolling onto my stomach once I am asleep?" he asked.

"One idea that seems to work is to place a tennis ball just above your belly button," I said. "Hold it in place with an elastic bandage, a sash from a robe, a scarf, or something similar. When you roll onto your stomach, you will feel the ball. It can 'knock the air out of you.' You will know it, 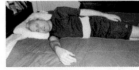 even in your sleep. You won't do it more than a couple of times before your brain will say, 'Nope, not going there.'"

I asked John why he sleeps on his stomach. "Always have," he said. "I'm so exhausted at the end of the day. I guess it's just a lazy way to fall into bed." As John and I discussed why he's so exhausted, he realized that he stays busy right up until he goes to bed. "I may spend some extra time on the computer at work and then try to get in a workout at the office gym before leaving. I often get home after the family has had dinner, so I eat while I watch the news. Sometimes I go to one of my kids' games before I go home, then I do my workout, grab fast food for dinner, finish my computer work at home, and later have a snack while I watch the news. This is after a full day in a stressful work environment. Yeah, I am pretty exhausted at night and can't wait to plop into bed."

"John," I said, "you need to slow down your mind and your body before you get so exhausted."

"How can I? There's always so much going on."

"How about a plan for your day and sleep routine?" Here are the suggestions I gave him:

- "If you go to your kid's game, how about choosing not to do any computer work at home that night?"
- "Maybe you don't need to listen to the news every night. That can give you a headache all by itself."
- "Look over your daily routine and occasionally choose to drop an activity or two."
- "Share some time with your wife or kids in the evening, just to relax and have fun."
- "Do some light stretching to relax your muscles before bedtime."
- "Go to bed a bit earlier."

As we reviewed what John considers his typical day, he realized he prefers doing things in the morning rather than late at night. He decided he could get up earlier and work out before going to the office, and occasionally even find time for his computer work in the morning. By listening to his body clock, John could have a less stressful day and still get to bed without being so exhausted. The choices he makes to diminish his fatigue, both mentally and physically, will allow him to choose a side or back sleep position, instead of just falling into bed on his stomach. John decided to better structure his day and be open to varying his schedule occasionally when work or home projects change. He also saw the value of taking some downtime in the evening to relax before going to bed. Together, these changes will reduce the muscle tension and strain that are contributing to John's headaches.

> **Other suggestions for dealing with stress:**
> *"If you are stressed...*
> *snack on Vitamin C and citrus fruits...*
> *it helps lower your cortisol, the stress hormone.*
> *Or instead of food, take a break, listen to music, or do*
> *something fun with friends."*
> —Mehmet Oz, M.D., host of *The Dr. Oz Show*

Randy. Randy came in later that day, complaining of headaches and a stiff neck when he slept. He remarked, "Sometimes my fingers tingle and sort of go numb. It gets better during the day but is always there at night. The worst is in the morning." Unlike John, Randy sleeps on his back with his arms above his head. A posture such as that shortens the neck and upper-back muscles, which can cause headaches as well as numbness in the arm and hand. I needed to take a closer look at his sleep posture and other factors that could be involved in Randy's pain.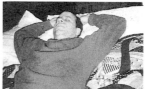

I had asked Randy to bring photographs of him sleeping and in daytime activities: sitting at his computer at home and at work, attending meetings, eating, reading, exercising, watching television, and even sitting in his car. Randy thought taking all those pictures was a little crazy. "No doctor or therapist has ever asked me for photographs," he said later as he handed me his photos. "But just looking at them, I can tell you aren't going to like them. I may not always be in the best posture, but I am not sure how all of this affects my headaches."

Randy's postures were affecting the same muscles in the neck and upper back that we identified earlier in John's postures. The same tight muscles were contributing to Randy's headaches. Randy's postures and work positions were different than John's, but shortened the same muscles.

Remember, what you do during the day *teaches* the muscles how you want them to function. Repeatedly shorten the muscles, and they will move to that position without any effort on your part: that is now their habit. That is how the muscles will work until you teach them something else. After looking at the way he sat at his computer, Randy said, "I have my shoulders hunched. Can that cause my headaches? I don't get it, it just seems so comfortable. I guess that's why it feels okay to have my arms up with my hands behind my head when I watch television at night and then when I go to bed."

As with John, tight muscles in Randy's neck and upper back were referring pain upward, resulting in headaches. Two shortened neck muscles were involved. Muscle (1) was pinching nerves in his neck and causing the numbness in his hands. Muscle (2) was responsible for Randy's waking with a stiff neck. Randy's challenge would be to keep his arms and shoulders down, in a more relaxed position, throughout the day. If he didn't change his current postures during the day, he would lie down and lapse into that same arms-up, pain-producing posture while he slept, and would continue waking with headaches and a stiff neck.

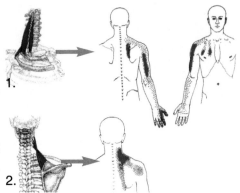

Randy commented, "This not-slouching thing is something I'm going to have to really consciously think about during the day. It isn't just going to happen. If I don't learn to sit up straight, with my arms and shoulders down and more relaxed, I'm going to keep doing it at night, and I'll never get rid of my headaches, will I?" A new habit—sitting up, butt to the back of the chair or sofa, and leaning against the back of the chair—was a must. This upright posture would bring his head over his shoulders and keep his hips, shoulders and ears in a straight line, allowing his neck muscles to relax and his shoulders to drop. Making these changes during the day would make it easier for his body to take the same alignment when he goes to bed.

Randy also realized that this new position had to be something he did regularly, not just part of the time. He would have to sit upright and learn to use the back of the chair consistently if it were to become a habit. The good news: the more often he uses the correct posture, the easier it will become, and the more responsive his body will be when lying down.

"Is there some way to make sure my arms stay down at night?" Randy asked.

"I have an odd but very effective way to help with that," I said. "Try sleeping in an oversized T-shirt, with your arms inside the shirt. Not like a straitjacket, just loose enough to allow a little movement, and just tight enough to keep your arms from going overhead." Randy laughed, but said he would try it.

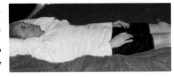

It took a night or two, but using this simple T-shirt solution, Randy "re-taught" his muscles to drop down to a regular, relaxed position, not hiked up around the ears, while he slept. The result: no more headaches, and no more arm and hand numbness, when he woke in the morning.

As we talked more about sleep positions, Randy mentioned something else that disturbed his sleep. "I get leg cramps at night. Since you figured out the headaches from the pictures I brought in, can you figure out the cramping, too?"

Dr. Janet Travell always said there were two ways to find the answer to a patient's pain:

- Check and recheck the pictures.
- Keep talking to your patient, listening and asking the right questions, and he or she will give you the answer.

Remembering her advice, Randy and I looked closely at his pictures again. We noticed the covers were pulled down tightly on his feet. This kept his toes pulled down, shortened his calf muscles, and could be causing his calf cramps.

"Randy," I said, "Untuck the covers at the bottom of your bed and put a pillow under the covers to hold them off your feet and toes. This will give your feet and legs room to move and relax, and it should help eliminate your leg cramps."

Randy closed our session saying, "It's amazing how such little changes in what I do during the day, and even at night, can eliminate the headaches, stiff neck, and leg cramps. No medications, no devices, just some common-sense changes. Guess it's knowing what to do and then choosing to make the changes that allow pain-free sleeping."

> *First say to yourself what you would be;*
> *then do what you have to do.*
> —Epictetus

Sandy. Sandy called the clinic and gave me a brief description of the back and hip pain that she experiences most evenings, which worsens as she sleeps. "I sleep on my side with my knees pulled up, and the top leg dropped over the bottom leg."

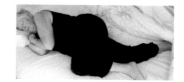

"Although it feels good, I realize it results in a distinct twisting of my hips and low back. In the morning, when I first get out of bed, it takes several minutes for me to work through the pain before I am able to stand upright. I really hope you can help me figure out what I can do. I am so tired of medications and exercises that either seem to do nothing or make it worse."

Once again, pictures were a key to discovering the answer to her pain. Sandy works in a garden center, at a job that requires constant bending forward, twisting, and turning. She frequently bends to trim plants and pot new ones, and twists as she reaches for planters, soil, and tools that are placed all around her. "I seem to be reaching and twisting all day long with my work, so I wouldn't think I would feel so tight at the end of work."

"Sandy," I explained, "you are bending, twisting, reaching, and turning a great deal, but it's often in a strained position, while you are lifting things at the same time. That kind of movement can be very stressful on the muscles, and it certainly is not a relaxed stretch that would eliminate tightness. Instead, the muscle continually shortens throughout the day."

Without stretching after work to remove the tightness from her muscles, Sandy heads home to fix dinner. Before starting, she often decides to take a quick nap. She does this while lying on the sofa on her side, knees up and hips twisted, with her top leg dropped over. This is a lying-down version of the torqued position she takes when standing at work. In preparing dinner, she will bend forward, twist, and turn at the counter, sink, and stove.

Sandy caught on as she looked at her photos and said, "Look at these pictures. I'm lying on the sofa on my side with one leg dropped way over the other one. That's exactly how I sleep at night. When I fix dinner, I'm in the same bending-forward and twisting positions I'm in all day at work. No wonder I sleep the way I do. I've been doing the same thing all day. My body is so used to it that it just goes there automatically."

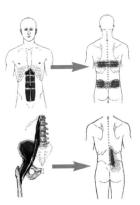

"Sandy," I said, "with your legs pulled up, you shorten a muscle that is right down the middle of your abdominal area, which produces pain across your low-back area." Most people think that where they *feel* pain is also the *origin* of the pain. Not so! Remember, it has been medically documented that shortness in an abdominal muscle shown here produces pain across the low-back area. Also, with your legs pulled up, you shorten a deeper muscle, also shown here, that flexes or bends your body at the hips. This documented pain referral pattern results in pain up and down in your low back.

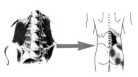

I explained further that one leg dropped over the other leg at night shortens this low-back muscle that results in hip pain. "Twisting during the day overuses this turning muscle, Sandy, and as tightness builds, it causes fatigue and pain. As a protection against additional strain, these muscles tighten even more. Doing this day after day, your muscles *learn* to function tight, or short. Remember, muscles will do whatever you teach them to do, right or wrong. They love it when you shorten them once again as you sleep on your side with your knees up, dropping your top leg over to twist your hips and low back. You're mimicking the bending forward and twisting of your daily life, and the muscles are responding with hip pain."

Sandy realized she needed to straighten out her body and her legs when she napped or slept. She couldn't change her work quite as easily, although she could reposition her tools and rearrange her work station so it was more convenient to maneuver without twisting and turning so much. She could also take breaks to stretch. She also thought she could vary her work tasks so she wasn't doing the same thing for extended periods and used different muscles. "And," she said, "no more curling up on the sofa in that twisted position for naps when I get home. I may just go for a short walk to get my body back in balance a little."

Thinking about what she was learning, Sandy asked a logical question. "I can change things at work and when I get home, but how can I change pulling my legs up and dropping one leg over the other when I'm asleep? Once I'm asleep, I don't know what I am doing. My legs just go where they always go."

"It may sound too simple," I responded, "but an easy aid is to put a big pillow in front of your body. The pillow acts as resistance when your legs start to pull up and keeps them extended. The pillow also gets in the way when you try to twist and drop your top leg over the bottom one."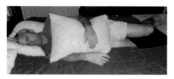

"Get into a side sleep position in the evening and lie on your bed holding the pillow for a couple of minutes, just to practice the new position. This will begin to prepare your body and mind for the real thing when you go to bed. After practicing and using the pillow for a few nights, you will re-teach your muscles to be longer and more relaxed. Your muscles will learn this new habit and will stay extended on their own."

"Sandy," I continued, "it's also useful to put a pillow between your knees. It helps keep your top leg from falling in front of the other and cushions your knees, too, so you won't feel like you have bone on bone. The pillow can be a full-sized bed pillow, or something more like a small pillow used in a chair or rocker. The pillow should extend from about six inches above the knee to at least six inches below the knee. It can extend down to the ankles and feet, if you like."

As Sandy and I continued to talk during her treatment session, she said to me, "I always feel cold when I go to bed, so I really pile on the covers. Does that make any difference in my pain?"

"Of course it could," I said. "If you're cold, that may be one of the reasons you tend to curl up as you go to sleep. Also, if you use a lot of covers, your muscles may be tensing against their weight. Why don't you set the heat just a little higher or try using an electric blanket? Turn it on to warm the bed before you get in, and then turn it off when you lie down."

"I have started using flannel sheets," Sandy offered. "They seem warmer than cotton ones, and I do feel like I relax a little more."

"Excellent!" I said. "We've put many pieces of your pain puzzle together. As you practice the changes and get comfortable with them, making them new habits, you will see your back and hip pain ease."

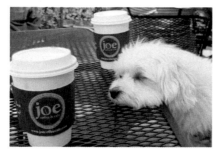

Sleep is always good; the positions may not always be the best!

Other Factors Affecting Sleep

Pillows

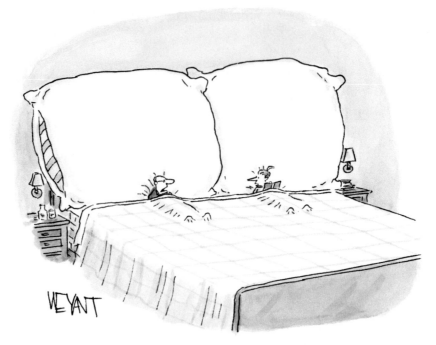

"Remember when all we had was lots of little pillows?"

Pick your pillows carefully.

Everyone should take seriously the choice of a pillow for sleeping. Pillows come in all shapes and sizes: flat, fat, round, skinny, wavy, bumpy, extra-long, and even tiny. One patient said, "I have a closet full of pillows but none of them really works. I've settled on one that feels 'kinda' okay, but not really."

How many pillows do you have stacked in your closet? You've tried them all, right? But you still wake up with a headache, a stiff neck, clenched jaw, dizziness, blurred vision, shoulder and chest pain, back pain, or even numbness and tingling down your arm. Could it be that you still don't have the pillow that's right for you? Or could it be that you don't know the best way to use your pillows?

Pillows need to be specific to you. They are not "one-size-fits-all." Each person is shaped differently, so you will need to find a pillow that fits you. The size of your head, how broad your shoulders are, how you sleep, even your hairstyle will determine the right type and size of pillow for *you*.

If you sleep on your back:

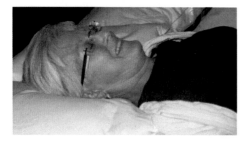

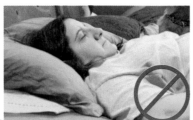

- Put a thin pillow behind your head.

- Pull the corners of the pillow in to fill the space under and around your neck.

- Make sure no part of the pillow is under your shoulder.

- The pillow should be thin enough under your head that it doesn't push your head forward and shorten muscles that could lead to a headache or stiff neck.

If you sleep on your side:

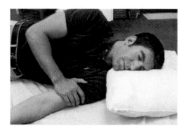

- Use a soft shredded or feather pillow to fill the space from your ear to the outside of your shoulder.

- The pillow should keep your head from tilting.

- If the pillow is too high, it will tilt your head sideways, and you can get a headache, a stiff neck, or numbness and tingling down your arm.

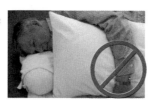

- If the pillow is too low, it may cause the same pain, but on the other side of your body.

- Have someone check your head position on the pillow.

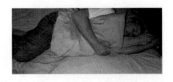

- Better yet, have someone take a picture so you can see your head position for yourself. Your head should be in line with your hip and shoulder, not out in front of them.

When you're shopping for a pillow, choose one that isn't solid foam. Some solid foam pillows can create extra motion as you move during the night, like a bowl of wiggling Jell-O. As a result, muscles tense and brace, trying to stabilize your body, and seldom relax completely. Other solid-foam materials hold your head so tightly that even incidental movement is restricted. Incidental movement during sleep helps to keep muscles loose. Your pillows should be filled with something pliable: shredded foam, feathers, or an alternative such as buckwheat kernels.

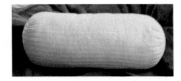

Tubular pillows, such as the original Jackson Cervipillo®, are designed to be softer in the center for back sleeping, since only a thin pillow is needed. The ends are firmer and provide good bulk for side sleeping.

Wedge pillows are not recommended for most people. Reading,watching television, or sleeping while propped up with a wedge pillow bends your body at the hips. Muscles are shortened in the front, as when you sleep on your side with your knees pulled up. To avoid the back and hip pain this posture can eventually produce, sleep flat with appropriate pillows. Sleeping on your side with a wedge pillow tends to jam the shoulder and tilt the head. This can result in a headache, stiff neck, arm and hand tingling, and stiff shoulders.

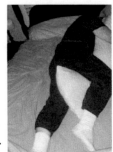

Body pillows tend to encourage you to wrap your leg up and over or around the pillow when you sleep on your side. You can experience the same back and hip pain we explored with Sandy earlier. If your arm drops over the pillow as well, you may experience shoulder and mid-back pain.

Choose a pillow that fits you. It's one more piece of the good-sleep puzzle.

Mattresses

Mattresses can make or break a good night's sleep. You can have a good sleep position and a perfect pillow, but with a lousy mattress you still don't get a good night's sleep, and you may often wake up experiencing muscle stiffness and pain.

- How old *is* your mattress? Ten years? Fifteen years? Even twenty years old? No amount of mattress flipping will help. Pillow tops or memory foam tops are fine, but of no use placed over an old mattress.

- Mattresses, like pillows, are not one-size-fits-all. They are an individual matter.

- A good mattress should allow you to assume a correct body position with the hip, shoulder, and ear in a straight line, and should also feel comfortable.

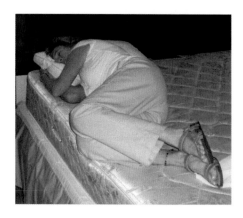

The shoulder is rolled
forward in front of the
hip, and the head is
even further forward

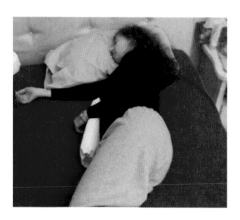

The hip, shoulder, and
ear are in a straight
alignment

- Don't let comfort be the only criterion in choosing a mattress. Remember, a bad position in bed may feel comfortable if it accommodates already tightened muscles.

- Lie on a mattress at the store for about twenty minutes and see if it's still comfortable.

- Many retailers will allow a thirty-day trial for the mattress. Don't hesitate to return it if it really isn't comfortable.

- Don't accept a mattress just because it's advertised to be the best. You're the one who has to sleep on it.

Beds

Beds come next. You've picked your pillow, tested your mattress, chosen your covers, and planned your sleep posture, but you still don't have a bed. Adjustable beds that put you into a semi-sitting position may look comfortable, but they're not suitable for teaching good muscle function. If the upper half of the bed is raised, your body is then in a slightly piked position, and several muscles in the front of your body are shortened. When you sleep on your side in a bed that is tilted, your side muscles are shortened. Back and hip pain can result.

If you need to have your bed elevated for a medical condition, Dr. Travell recommended simply elevating the head of the bed about three and one-half inches by placing a brick sideways under the legs at the head of the bed. You can also purchase bed risers for this purpose. This slight incline of the head of the bed exerts mild natural traction on the body while you sleep, keeping the head higher than the rest of your body. Lying in such a nice, gradual incline, your body tends to be more relaxed, without the need for "trying to get comfortable."

Summary

The pain experienced by the patients we discussed, John, Randy, and Sandy, had similar components:

- Postures at work and home
- Furniture
- Stresses
- The need to stretch

By making small changes and practicing them, they have allowed their bodies to function in a more balanced and natural way. Making *habits* of these changes helps eliminate pain. The following section on sleep postures will help you identify incorrect positions you may be using, so you can fix them and begin to enjoy relief from pain. When you choose to make changes to eliminate pain, allowing you a restful, satisfying, rejuvenating night's sleep, you'll find your energy and zest for life returning.

> *If you get the inside right,*
> *the outside will fall*
> *into place.*
> —Eckhart Tolle

Posture Evaluation and Correction

"CURLED" POSTURE

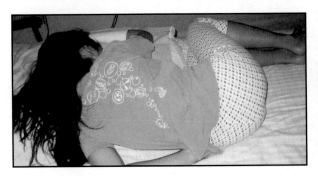 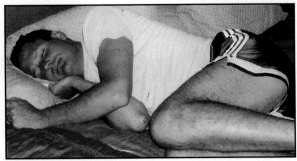

Wow! How do I straighten up from this curl without stiffness and pain?

Why is it so comfortable, if it causes all this pain?

Muscles do what we teach them. They tighten from normal, everyday use, and they relax or loosen with stretching. If the muscles are not stretched regularly during the day, tension remains in the muscles, and they begin to feel *normal* in this *learned short* position. You then accommodate the muscle shortness so it even begins to *feel good* as you sleep *curled.* Comfortable does not always mean correct, however. Tight muscles often result in pain.

Note the muscles involved in sleeping *curled* and the pain that results from the tightness in those muscles:

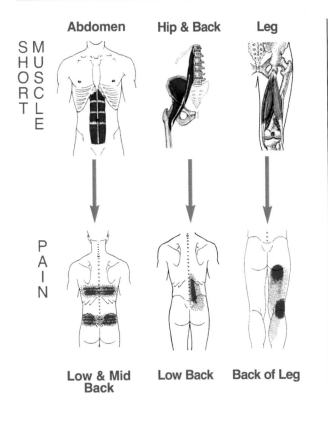 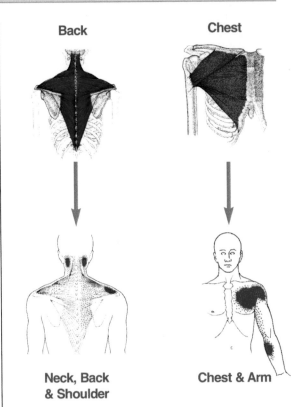

New sleep posture habits help you to wake without pain.

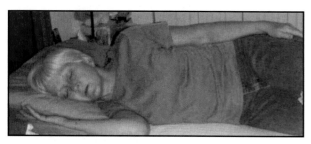

Corrected "Curled" Posture

Sleep postures that you take at night are usually learned from postures you use during the day, and vice versa. Changing to good alignment, both sitting and standing, will be reinforced with your sleep posture, for a quicker elimination of your pain.

"Change such old habits when I am asleep?" Here's how:

1 **Become a pillow hugger**
Once you are asleep, a pillow in front of your body will act as a slight resistance if you try to pull your legs toward your chest. Placing your arm by your side, with your forearm on the pillow, keeps your shoulder down and prevents you from dropping your arm in front of your body.

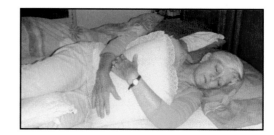

2 **Place a pillow between your knees**
A pillow between your knees helps keep both legs in a more extended position, not allowing one leg to drop in front of the other leg. It also provides a cushion between the knees.

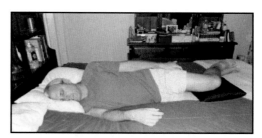

3 **Practice before bedtime**
Practice this new position several times during the evening, just for a minute or two. This prepares the brain, body, and muscles to assume the position during sleep. It will take only a few nights for it to become comfortable, and a new habit.

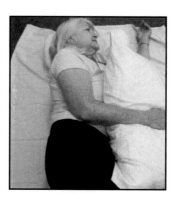

4 **Stretch**

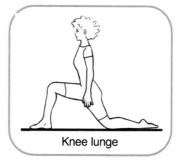

Knee lunge

STRETCHING begins to lengthen your shortened muscles, teaching them to stay in a more relaxed, extended position when you are asleep. This new posture then establishes *new muscle memory* and *muscle habits* that keep muscles from taking incorrect postures, leaving you free from muscle pain.

Stretch your way to pain-free activity

> **Stretches change muscle function.**

Stretch to bring the muscles to a resting and balanced position to teach them a new way to function and allow movement without pain.

Stretching can be integrated into your daily activities without the need for a special place or time. Some stretches can be performed while waiting at a red light or taking a phone call. Performed throughout the day, for just a minute or two, stretching can make the difference between having chronic aches and pains, and being free to live life.

> **Not stretching muscles allows tightness to build, resulting in aches and pains. Stretching releases the tightness, eliminating pain.**

The stretches on the next page will shift your tight muscles to a more elongated and relaxed position. You'll be more comfortable in sleep and will avoid waking in pain. Anyone can take a minute to stretch. The difference in muscle comfort is awesome.

The Rule of Two for Stretching

2 — Repetitions:	Complete two repetitions of each stretch.
2 — Breaths:	Hold each stretch for two breaths before releasing.
2 — Hours:	Repeat each stretch every two hours to develop *new muscle memory.*
2 — Sides:	Stretch both sides of the body, but just one side at a time, to gain balance throughout the body.

FOCUS
- **This** is a *feel-good* stretch, not a *see-how-far-you-can-push* stretch.
- **Feel** a slight stretch, avoiding a hard pull.
- **Hold** each stretch position gently. It should feel comfortable.
- **Make** the stretch a smooth movement, without any bouncing.
- **Everything** should be as relaxed as possible when you stretch.

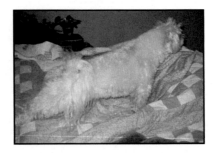

Stretches specific for reversing the muscle tightness from *curled* sleeping

Stretches are numbered in the order designed to best balance the muscles. If you are in a situation where you cannot do the floor stretches, do the standing ones. All of the stretches should be performed at home. Many people are able to find a place at work to do all of the stretches, too.

1.

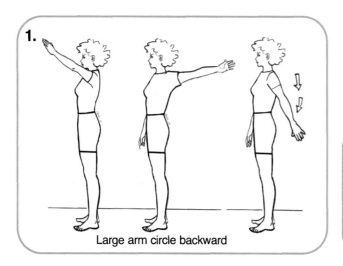

Large arm circle backward

2.

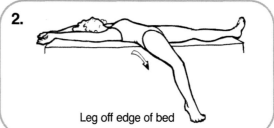

Leg off edge of bed

3.

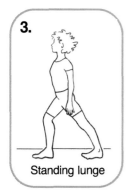

Standing lunge

4.

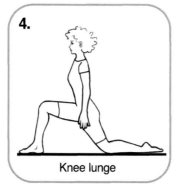

Knee lunge

5.

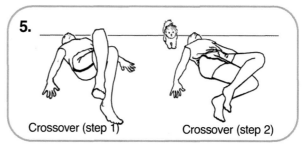

Crossover (step 1)   Crossover (step 2)

6.

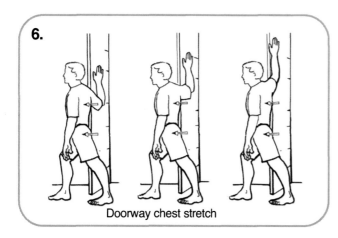

Doorway chest stretch

7.

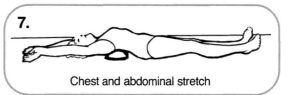

Chest and abdominal stretch

Please refer to *Appendix 1: Stretch Instructions* in the back of this book for more details on these stretches.

"SIDEWINDER" POSTURE

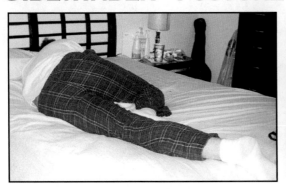
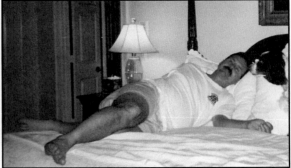

Yikes! This twisted sleep posture produces painful results:

- Knees, back, hips, and legs experience considerable strain, as shown below.
- Notice the pain, shown below, in the arms, shoulders, neck, and head as well.

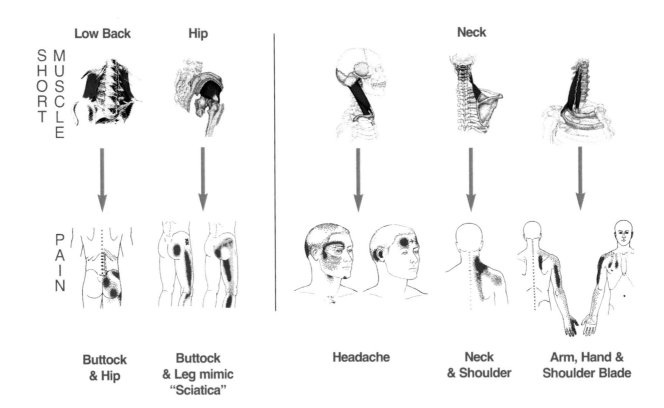

The postures you assume when sleeping indicate what you have taught your muscles to do throughout the day. The challenge is to teach them during the day to be elongated and balanced in a way that allows you to sleep restfully and pain free at night.

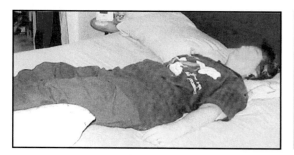
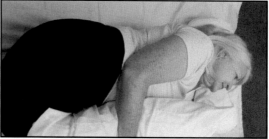

Corrected "Sidewinder" Posture

Aligning the center of the hip, shoulder, and ear in a straight, neutral position encourages pain-free sleeping.

"Once I'm asleep, my body just goes the wrong way. How do I change that?"

1

Put a large pillow in front of you
Place the pillow in front of the body to hug. This will help keep the body from twisting. Hugging the pillow also keeps the shoulders from shrugging and helps keep the head from rolling forward.
Hip – shoulder – ear in a straight line = no pain

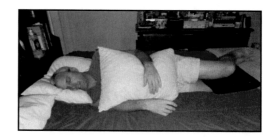

2

Put a small pillow between your knees
A pillow between your knees helps keep both legs in a more elongated position, not allowing one leg to easily drop in front of the other. It also provides a cushion between the knees. *Note:* the pillow is just above the knees but may extend further down the legs to the feet.

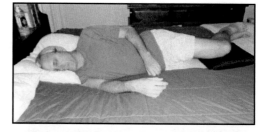

3

Practice before bedtime
Practice the new sleep posture for a minute or two in the evening to prepare the brain, body and muscles for sleep. It will only take a few nights for the new posture to become a *habit*.

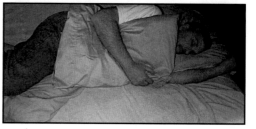

Your tight muscles are the *why* of your chronic pain. Stretching and relaxation allow a new, elongated pattern of muscle function that does not result in pain.

Learn about stretching on the following pages will help you teach the muscles this new way of functioning.

Stretch and relax

Stretching and relaxation put you in control.

Stretching and relaxation can become something you look forward to. Don't let yourself neglect to take care of of your body, no matter how busy you may be. You put tension in your muscles all day long just from using them. All they ask is that you occasionally stop, take some deep breaths, and do a couple of stretches. This takes only a few minutes. At the end of the day, you will have used a total of fifteen to twenty minutes. Everyone is worth taking those few minutes to allow the muscles to release tension and function freely and without pain.

Good stretch habits = No pain and restful sleep

Learn stretches that are the opposite of the type of movement you do at work and throughout the day. For example, if you bend forward frequently during your work, your stretches should move your body backward. This might include large arm circles backward or taking a forward/backward step position and then reaching the arms overhead. If you lift or reach while twisting and turning only in one direction, your stretches should be overhead reaching and twisting in the opposite direction.

Many stretches you see here may seem contrary to what you have previously thought you should do. Look closely at the muscles you are stretching, not necessarily where you feel discomfort.

- **Low-back pain** requires stretching the abdominal and hip muscles by leaning backward.
- **Temple headaches** require stretching the top of the shoulders downward.
- **Knee pain** needs stretching the muscles in the front of the upper leg backward.

The stretches on the next page will shift your short muscles from the *sidewinder* sleep posture to longer, balanced, and more relaxed positions. These new postures can become new *muscle habits* that allow you to experience pain-free sleep.

Follow these simple rules when performing your stretches.

Stretch to relax.

The Rule of Two for Stretching

2 — **Repetitions:**	Complete two repetitions of each stretch.
2 — **Breaths:**	Hold each stretch for two breaths before releasing.
2 — **Hours:**	Repeat each stretch every two hours to develop *new muscle memory.*
2 — **Sides:**	Stretch both sides of the body, but just one side at a time, to gain balance throughout the body.

Stretching requires only a slight pull and no bouncing.
Feel-good stretching requires all muscles to be as relaxed as possible.

Stretches for reversing the muscle tightness that resulted from *sidewinder* sleeping

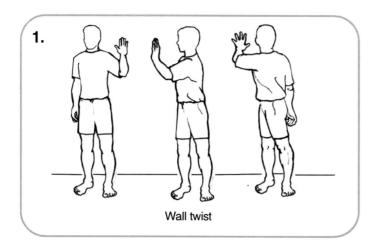

1.

Wall twist

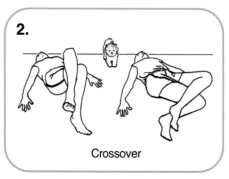

2.

Crossover

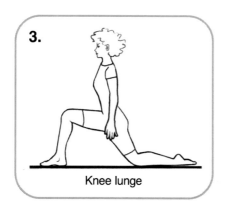

3.

Knee lunge

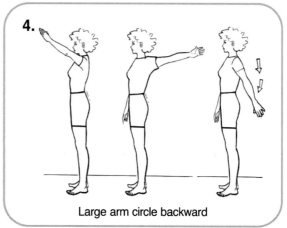

4.

Large arm circle backward

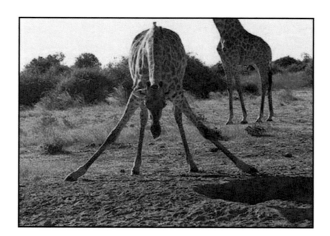

"STOMACH SLEEPING" POSTURE

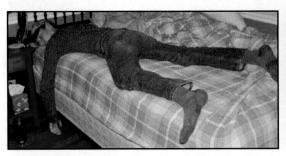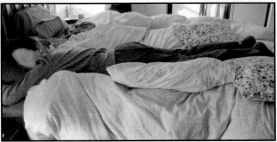

Ouch! Stomach sleeping is a posture that leads to pain. Turning the head to one side and lifting the shoulders results in a stiff neck, headaches, and arm and hand numbness and tingling.

Sleeping on my stomach really *feels good*. How can that be bad?

Stomach sleeping feels like a snug, secure sleep posture. Have you noticed, however, that what *feels good* isn't always good for you? Postures that repeatedly shorten muscles during the day will be mimicked at night, since that is what muscles have *learned* to do. Short muscles eventually result in pain.

Toes pointed and feet turned out can result in knee, calf, and foot pain; cramping, and plantar fasciitis.

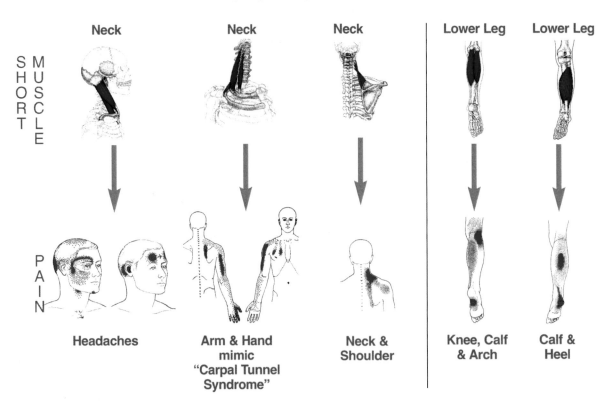

	Neck	Neck	Neck	Lower Leg	Lower Leg
SHORT MUSCLE					
PAIN	Headaches	Arm & Hand mimic "Carpal Tunnel Syndrome"	Neck & Shoulder	Knee, Calf & Arch	Calf & Heel

Taking these new sleep positions can make waking up feel good!

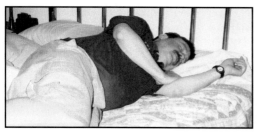

Corrected "Stomach Sleeping" Posture

Modify the *stomach* posture by sleeping on your side or back. A straight head position and relaxed, neutral foot position helps eliminate pain during sleep.

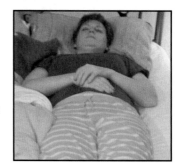

How can I change such old and comfortable postures when I am asleep?

Use a tennis ball
Place a tennis ball, secured by a an elastic bandage, just above your belly button. When you turn on your stomach, the pressure of the ball will knock the air out of you. Do it a couple of times, and the brain won't let you do it again.

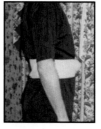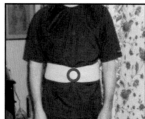

Become a pillow hugger
Once you are asleep, the pillow acts as a slight resistance to your rolling forward onto your stomach and pulling your leg up.

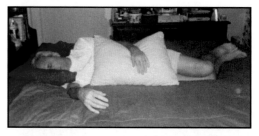

Use pillow support
Use a thin pillow behind your head. Pull the ends around your neck to help keep the head from rolling side to side.

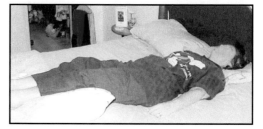

Stretch

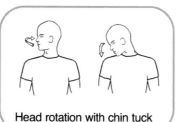

Head rotation with chin tuck

Once you become used to your new sleep posture, stretching will teach your muscles to accept working in this new position. Consistently using the new postures will teach new *muscle habits* that do not elicit pain.

Please refer to *Appendix 1: Stretch Instructions* in the back of this book for more details on these stretches.   **45**

Stretching is next

Stretching should be an integral part of your day. You constantly use your muscles causing tension to build up. You need to stretch the muscles frequently if they are to remember the elongated postures that allow you to enjoy a restful night of sleep.

> **Fill a muscle with enough tension or shortness, and it will eventually be too tight to work effectively. Cramping, fatigue, weakness, stiffness, and pain can result.**

Make stretching a natural part of your day. You do not need a specific time or place, or even a lot of time, to accomplish more elongated muscles.

Use 30 seconds for stretching:
- when you get out of bed or finish your shower
- when waiting for the bus, or ride to work; or when you get in and out of your car

Use 15 seconds for stretching:
- when you get up from your desk
- at lunch time or during coffee breaks
- when waiting for the elevator
- when waiting in a line shopping

The Rule of Two for Stretching

2 — **Repetitions:**	Complete two repetitions of each stretch.	
2 — **Breaths:**	Hold each stretch for two breaths before releasing.	
2 — **Hours:**	Repeat each stretch every two hours to develop *new muscle memory*	
2 — **Sides:**	Stretch both sides of the body, but just one side at a time, to gain balance throughout the body.	

FOCUS

- **This** is a *feel-good* stretch, not a *see-how-far-you-can-push* the stretch.
- **Feel** a slight stretch, avoiding a hard pull.
- **Hold** each stretch position gently. It should feel comfortable.
- **Make** the stretch a smooth movement, without any bouncing.
- **Everything** should be as relaxed as possible when you stretch.

Stretches for reversing the muscle tightness resulting from *stomach sleeping*

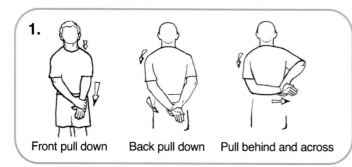

1. Front pull down   Back pull down   Pull behind and across

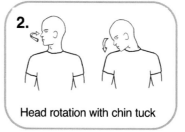

2. Head rotation with chin tuck

Do all of the stretches in the order shown.

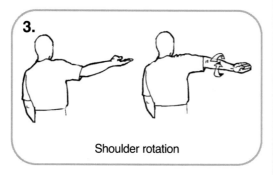

3. Shoulder rotation

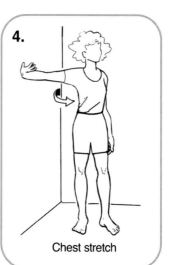

4. Chest stretch

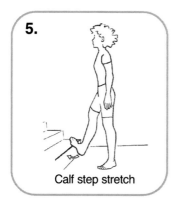

5. Calf step stretch

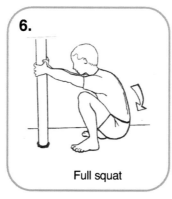

6. Full squat

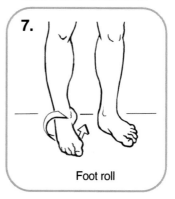

7. Foot roll

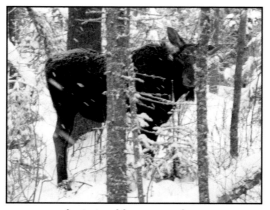

Just streching my neck.

Please refer to **Appendix 1: Stretch Instructions** in the back of this book for more details on these stretches.

"ARMS UP" POSTURE

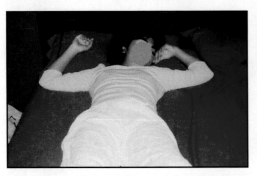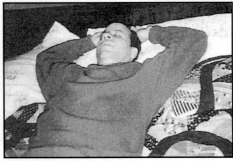

Oh no! The arms raised in surrender will certainly result in morning pain.
Here's why.

The arms raised shorten the upper back, shoulder, and neck muscles; and strain the mid-back muscles = pain. Check out the pain patterns below to see some of the pain you can experience.

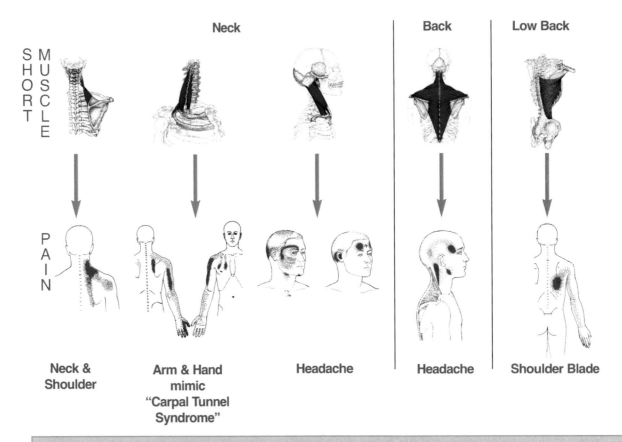

	Neck			Back	Low Back

SHORT MUSCLE

PAIN

| Neck & Shoulder | Arm & Hand mimic "Carpal Tunnel Syndrome" | Headache | Headache | Shoulder Blade |

**"All of this pain because I have my arms overhead when I sleep?
That seems extreme."**

While it doesn't seem like much, the arms overhead pull hard on the chest and some of the upper-back muscles. This position also shortens, or jams up, the top of the arms, shoulders, and neck muscles. Both the strain of the pull on some muscles, and the shortening of the others, can result in significant pain.

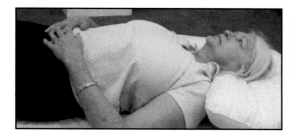
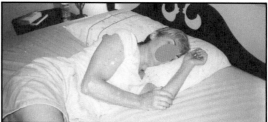

Corrected "Arms Up" Posture

You may wonder how you can be sure your arms are down if you are sound asleep?

Whether sleeping on your stomach or back, your arms have to come down to eliminate your pain. Stomach sleeping is undesirable, so you need to find a workable back or side position. Here are some good options:

Use an oversized T-shirt
Place your arms inside a loose oversized T-shirt when sleeping on your back. This makes it difficult for the arms to reach overhead.

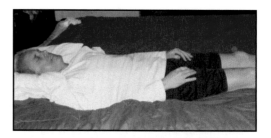

Use a sash
Loosely tying a bathrobe sash around your waist and around the wrists limits arm movement, not allowing the arms to reach above the head. You can also lie on the sash with the ends tied loosely around the wrists.

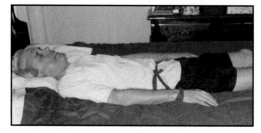

Use your own body resistance
Place your arms at your side, with some of your fingers tucked under your buttock. The slight pressure on your hand will act as a resistance to lifting the arms overhead.

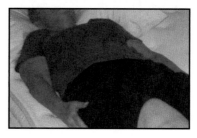

Practice before bedtime to prepare your mind and body for success

To be successful quickly, follow the stretch program on the following pages. The simplicity of the stretches is most effective in releasing muscle tension and in allowing the muscles to relax.

Stretching, the final key to success

> **Okay, you have mastered the sleep posture, now what? Stretch!**

"What is the big deal with stretching? I usually stretch before a workout, sometimes even in the morning. That should be good, right?"

Not quite! If you want the muscles to function from a loose position, not all shortened up, you have to teach them something different than what they have been doing. If you stretch only once a day, even for 30 minutes, but the rest of the day the muscles are on their own, they will just return to what they know = short.

If you want to learn to play a new sport, work out to lose weight, or learn another language, you don't just spend a few minutes a day, and then forget about it until some other convenient time. No, you learn what you have to do, and you practice, practice, practice. Then you see the results.

The Rule of Two for Stretching

2 — Repetitions: Complete two repetitions of each stretch.
2 — Breaths: Hold each stretch for two breaths before releasing.
2 — Hours: Repeat each stretch every two hours to develop *new muscle memory*.
2 — Sides: Stretch both sides of the body, but just one side at a time, to gain balance throughout the body.

F O C U S

- **This** is a *feel-good* stretch, not *see-how-far-you-can-push* stretch.
- **Feel** a slight stretch, avoiding a hard pull.
- **Hold** the stretch position gently.
- **Make** the stretch a smooth movement, without any bouncing.
- **Everything** should be as relaxed as possible when you stretch.

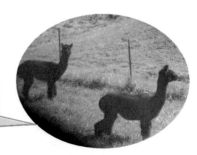

Come on, we're suppose to stretch.

Stretches specifically designed for reversing the muscle tightness resulting from *arms-up* sleeping

Do these stretches in the order given for balanced movement in your muscles.

These stretches are easy to do, and you need to do only 2 repetitions every 2 hours. Simplicity and frequency are what makes them work. Be nice to yourself, and reverse your chronic pain.

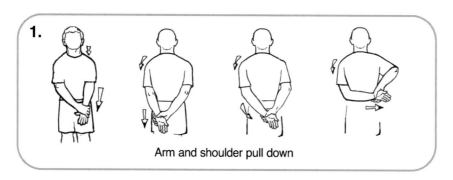

1.

Arm and shoulder pull down

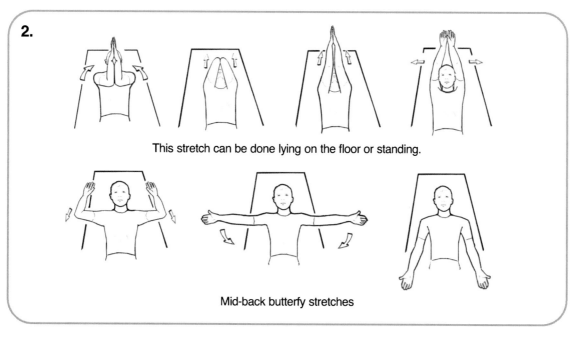

2.

This stretch can be done lying on the floor or standing.

Mid-back butterfy stretches

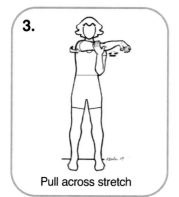

3.

Pull across stretch

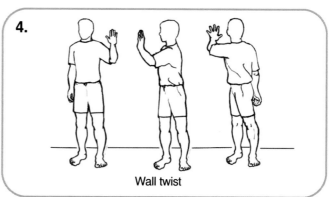

4.

Wall twist

"HALF SIDE, HALF STOMACH" POSTURE

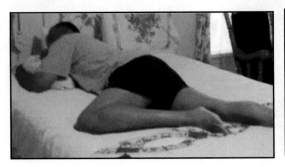 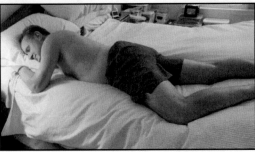

Help! This combination of side, stomach, and head-turned sleeping is a position that will result in pain.

"Isn't it normal to take a really comfortable position so you can get to sleep easily? What's wrong with that?"

Remember, *comfortable is not always correct.* The postures you use during the day are what make this position comfortable at night. It will be important to change your daytime postures so the body does not try to mimic a bad *muscle habit* when you sleep.

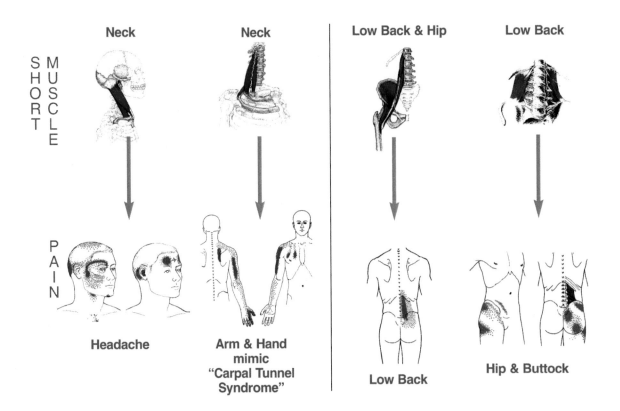

SHORT MUSCLE

| Neck | Neck | Low Back & Hip | Low Back |

PAIN

Headache | Arm & Hand mimic "Carpal Tunnel Syndrome" | Low Back | Hip & Buttock

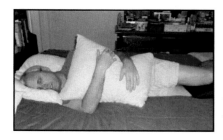

Moving to a neutral position that puts the center of your hip, shoulder, and ear in a straight line will allow muscles to relax while you sleep, relieving tightness and pain.

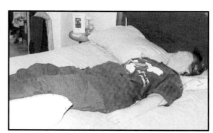

Corrected "Half side, Half Stomach" Posture

This is crazy. How can I change how I sleep when I am asleep?

You will need some props to help you make changes in your sleep posture. Otherwise, you will move to your usual position as soon as you are asleep. Here are some suggestions:

Use a tennis ball
Secure a tennis ball just above your belly button with a sash or cloth belt, just tight enough to hold it in place. If you roll onto your stomach, you will wake up as the ball knocks the air out of you. Do this a few times, and the brain won't let it happen again.

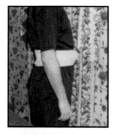 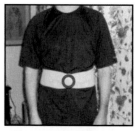

Become a pillow hugger
If you are going to side sleep, you need something in front of your body to keep you from rolling forward. A regular big bed pillow works well. Hugging the pillow keeps the arms down, and its position in front of your body acts as a resistance to raising your leg.

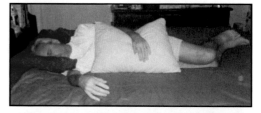

Choose your back
For back sleeping, use a thin pillow under your head and a small pillow under your knees. You can even try placing a big pillow beside you to make it more difficult to roll onto your side and stomach.

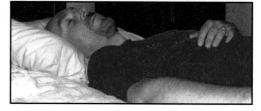

Practice before bedtime
Practice the new sleep posture a couple of times in the evening. Do a few stretches to help relax your muscles and remove unwanted tension.

Follow the stretch program on the following pages to begin a new level of function with your muscles. A simple approach to stretching has been designed to help eliminate your pain.

Stretch to feel good

Stretch Numbers: **2 Repetitions** — too many repetitions can fatigue muscles instead of teaching new *muscle memory.*

Stretch Duration: **2 Breaths** — taking a couple of deep breaths relaxes the muscles, resulting in less pain.

Stretch Frequency: **2 Hours** — frequency teaches muscles what you want them to do, instead of muscles reverting to old patterns of being tight.

Stretch Areas: **2 Sides** — both sides create a balance throughout the body.

F

O

C

U

S

Make stretching fun by stretching gently. There is no need for a hard stretch. You are trying to undo muscle tension, not win a contest.

Feel only a slight pull on the muscle, take a deep breath, and increase the range of stretch just slightly on the exhale. Try that again, just one more time, before moving on to another stretch.

Once you reach the light pull or stretch, hold the position steady, avoiding bouncing or moving about. In this held position, the muscle *learns* where you want it to function. You actually teach it how you want it to move.

When you do your stretches, relax all of your muscles as much as possible. There is no need to posture when stretching: putting your hands on your hips or holding your head up when you are bending forward. You are trying to teach your muscles to relax when they are not working. It is difficult to take deep breaths and relax into a stretch when you are being tight or stiff in another part of the body.

Let stretch *feel good.* Learn to turn off all those thoughts whirling around in your head, and for just a couple of minutes, just *be,* just *relax.*

> **Take your time when stretching. Feel your body relax.**

54

Stretches specifically chosen for reversing the muscle tightness from *half-side, half-stomach* sleeping

- Do these stretches in the order given when you are at home.
- Do just the standing stretches if you are away from home and not in a situation where you can easily do stretches on the floor. You may be able to find a place at work to do floor stretches.

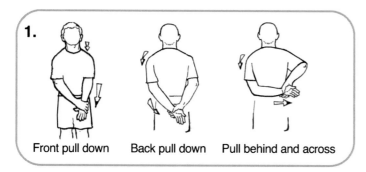

1.

Front pull down   Back pull down   Pull behind and across

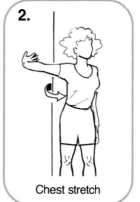

2.

Chest stretch

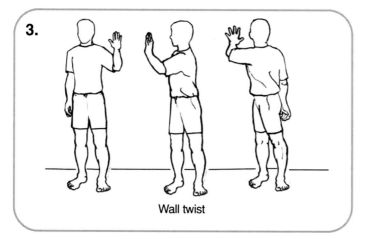

3.

Wall twist

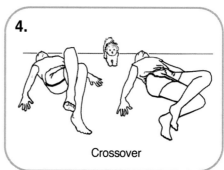

4.

Crossover

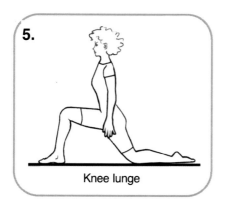

5.

Knee lunge

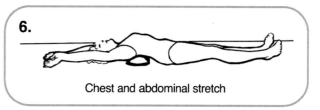

6.

Chest and abdominal stretch

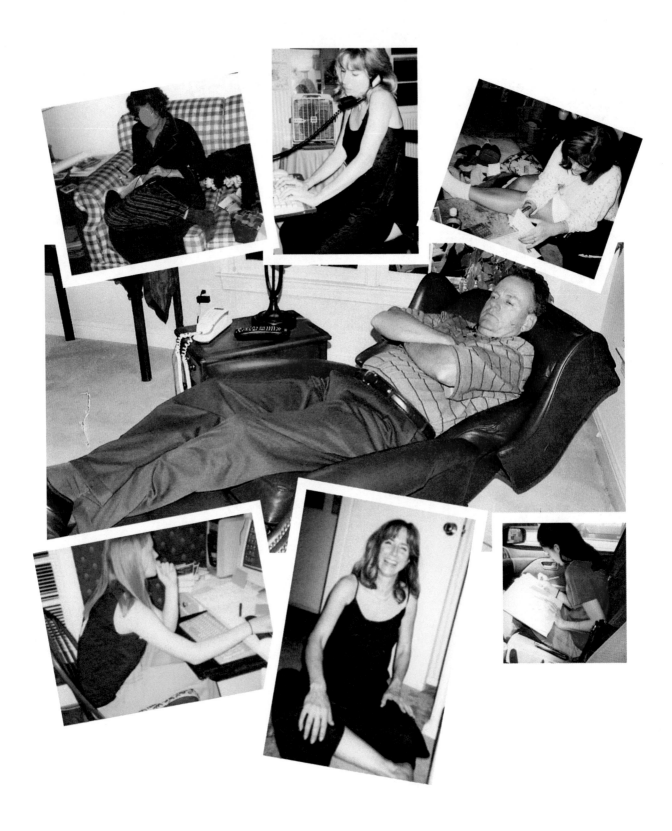

Chapter 3.
Sitting: Pain Instead of Relaxation

*S*itting. You wouldn't think it would be so hard to get it right. We sit all the time at work, home, and play. It certainly is not difficult to get comfortable; just watch people settle into a chair, sofa, or recliner. Oh, but remember—comfortable *is not always good for you.*

The following scenarios are taken from discussions I had with patients who came to my clinic for help with chronic pain they believed came from sitting.

Mark. Mark walked into my clinic one day. His friends, former patients of mine, had tried to get him to address his back pain for months. "I thought it would get better if I gave it time. It just seems to be getting worse, so I thought I had better get some help," he said. "It used to hurt only when I was getting up from a chair or sofa. Now sitting itself, anywhere, for any length of time at all, is really painful."

We scheduled a consultation and talked briefly about what he should bring with him. I asked that someone take photographs of him in all his sitting postures: reading, watching television, working at the computer, eating, and from the side, sitting in the car. I also wanted pictures of all of his sleep postures. Those could be taken at any time, even during the day. The pictures would show us what Mark is doing with his muscles as he goes about his day, and what might be causing his pain.

Mark came for his consultation to review the pictures and talk about activities, work, stresses, and hobbies that might be causing or perpetuating his pain.

Mark's description of his pain focused on a band of pain across the low back and another band across his mid back. He mentioned that he also had pain in the low back that tended to go up and down along his spine. Groin and hip pain occasionally crept in as well.

I explained to Mark that it is common for a major source of back and groin pain to be from muscles located in the front of the body.

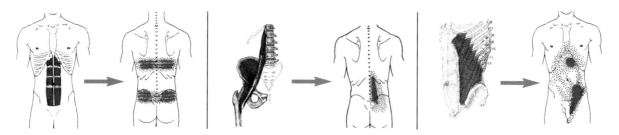

These muscles are shortened repeatedly from the bending that is done with so many daily activities. Mark was bending forward almost from the time he got up until he went to bed: brushing his teeth, shaving, eating, getting dressed, and tying his shoes. Mark's bending and rounding his back continued at work as he sat at his desk and attended meetings. Once he got home in the evening, he kept the same posture as he did routine tasks like paying bills, checking the computer, or helping with homework.

"I play golf, too, so that means I bend forward more often than some folks," he remarked.

"That's a good insight, Mark, and you'll probably think of other things you do during the day that put you in that bent or rounded posture. A rounded position always puts the muscles in the front of the hips and torso in a shortened and stressed position, contributing to your back pain. Let's take a look at your pictures and see what else we notice," I said.

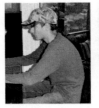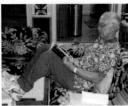

A quick glance revealed Mark often sits at his computer leaning forward, both at work and at home. "Mark, look at this. You take the same bent-forward, rounded posture when you are relaxing or lounging on the sofa in the evening as you do at your computer. Only now your feet are propped up on the coffee table as you slouch. You keep the same muscles shortened, you've just changed locations." Shortened abdominal and hip bending muscles result from this rounded back. In fact, Mark's hips are bent even more with his feet propped up, adding to his back pain.

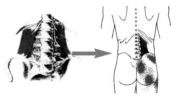

Mark's *propped up* and *slouch* postures continued as he watched television in bed.Now, however, he added a twist—literally. He had to twist a little to see the television that was placed in the corner of the room. His torqued posture stressed and shortened a low-back muscle that is responsible for a lot of hip pain.

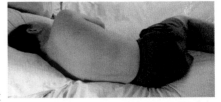

As we continued to look at the pictures, the sleep postures caught our attention. "Mark," I explained, "you sit forward and rounded at work and at home, and add bending forward with golf. You take those postures so frequently it is no wonder your muscles continue to be comfortable in a "curled" sleep position at night." The reinforcement of *teaching* your muscles to stay short during the night; the added rounded-back and slouched sitting during the day results in constant pain. You start with shortened muscles when you get up in the morning, then all the bending forward during the day builds more tension to the point where the muscles can't handle any more contraction, and they inevitably talk back with pain.

"The good news," I said, "is there are postural changes you can make quite easily. Give me your thoughts on a few simple guidelines you might follow."

"Okay, here goes," he said. "First, I do sit with my butt all the way back in my chair and on the sofa but I guess I need to lean back also, instead of leaning forward and slouching. That would do away with the rounded back, wouldn't it? That probably goes for any place I sit, right?"

"Yes," I replied. "Think of aligning the center of your hip, center of your shoulder, and ear in a straight line as you sit. This allows your spine and your chair to help support you, instead of straining muscles to sit upright."

"And I can rearrange my furniture so the television is in front of me instead of off to the side," Mark continued. "That eliminates tightening the twisting and turning muscles that give me the hip pain, but I still need to sit up straight. I think I am beginning to get this posture thing, but I am really going to have to focus on it instead of just plopping down in a chair."

"Place all of your furniture or projects directly in front of you: television, computer, hobbies, reading, gardening, and so forth. Eliminate the torqued or turned posture to keep your hip and low-back muscles looser and balanced," I emphasized.

"I really need to get a new sofa that is a lot firmer," he concluded. "The one I have is way too soft. I've known that, but just haven't gotten around to picking out a new one."

It was only a few days before Mark called to give me the results of his efforts to buy new furniture and change his sitting posture. "You won't believe how much better my pain is already, just from making the posture changes we talked about. Well, I guess you would believe it," he chuckled. I still fall back into old sitting postures occasionally, but I catch myself right away. I guess it's like anything else, the more I practice the right posture, the better I feel."

> **All motion is easier
> when muscles move with total freedom.**

> **You do not need to see far ahead;
> just one step at a time
> accomplishes your goal.**

Lacy. Sitting, especially for any length of time, caused a lot of headaches for Lacy. Because of the pain, she was missing work and was not enjoying life.

"I sure hope you can help me. Besides missing work and not having much of a social life, I also have two little ones at home who demand a lot of time and attention," Lacy sighed. Her children are very active three- and five-year olds, so she expends a lot of energy keeping up with them.

"Lacy, how about bringing in photographs of your most frequent sitting situations: eating, playing with the kids, sitting at your computer at home and at work, at your desk working on projects or on phone conference calls, a side view of you in your car, and a couple of you relaxing after the kids are in bed," I suggested. "We really need to put all the pieces in front of us to figure out what is causing your headaches."

"It may take a while to get the pictures, as my husband does a lot of traveling with his work," she said. "Or perhaps I could get my neighbor to take them. She's become a good friend since we moved in."

Lacy was a few minutes late arriving for her appointment later that week and looked exhausted. "My headache is particularly bad today. One of the children was up a lot during the night, and both of them were fussy at breakfast. Then the babysitter was late, and the office called just as I was about to walk out the door. Way too much going on, right now!" Lacy said. "Not only do I hope you can help, but I sure hope the solution isn't too complicated, because I just don't have much energy left."

As Lacy took a moment to relax with a cup of tea, we began to visit and to identify factors in her day that contributed to her headaches. Many of her postures during the day shortened and stressed muscles in her neck and shoulders. These muscles are often the very ones responsible for headaches. We decided to take a few minutes to see what postural situations Lacy could identify what she thought shortened her muscles. We then worked on solutions for them.
Her list included the following situations, along with suggested solutions.

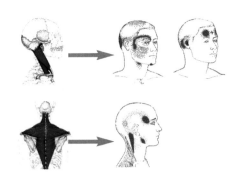

Muscle Shortening Occurs	*Suggested Solutions*
• Sitting on the floor playing games with the children	• Bring the games to a table or higher surface, making sure everyone has an appropriate chair.
• Reading to the children while sitting on the edge of their beds with no support	• Place a chair close the bed for myself, so I can still share the book and pictures easily.
• Eating, always bending, reaching, and helping one of the kids	• Consider having the children use a booster chair, if necessary. Allow them to take their own servings at meals.
• Dressing the children, again bending and reaching	• Lay out their clothes and allow them to help dress themselves. Be patient as they learn to do this. Squat in front of them or sit in a chair to do zippers.
• Taking a quick sit-down without sitting square at the computer	• If it is a quick sit-down, perhaps it is best to wait until later.
• Multi-tasking at work: computer, phone, and writing, generally rounding my posture	• Intentionally break up my work rather than always trying to multi-task. Some things really can wait.
• Sitting slouched at work, just trying to relax	• Take a five-minute walk to clear my head and move my muscles.
• Eating at my desk while still working on something	• Decide not to do this. Bring lunch and go to the lunch room, or go out to eat. I need the break anyway.
• Plopping in the recliner to watch television after the kids are in bed	• Ill-fitting furniture or floppy postures increase muscle tension. Make furniture fit so I can truly relax. Breathe deeply.
• Tilting the car seat back so the headrest doesn't hit my head, but then I am leaning backward and my head is forward	• Put a small pillow behind my back at waist height to help me sit more upright, while leaving my head free of the seat's headrest.

"Whew, what a list!" I said. "I almost get a headache just looking over all you have going on. I think many of the suggestions will be helpful to you and allow you to enjoy the children while being less stressed at work and at home. Remember, also, that sugary foods are comfort foods. Don't let yourself fall into the habit of eating poorly when you are stressed."

"Let's give these alternatives a try and see how it goes," I continued. "Give me a call in a few days, and remember, children will adapt more easily to the changes if they are still having a good time with you and are even getting to try some new things. It seems adults have the more difficult time making changes, perhaps because they have forgotten to have fun along the way."

Other suggestions for dealing with stress, anxiety, or feeling overwhelmed:

- Avoid refined sugar. It may give a quick jolt of energy, but it won't last when the blood levels inevitably crash and you are left feeling irritated and exhausted.

- Stay hydrated. A small study in the *Journal of Nutrition* showed that being just over one percent below optimal hydration levels can result in headaches, loss of focus, and fatigue.
  —Mehmet Oz, M.D., host of *The Dr. Oz Show*

Sitting—more ways than you can count. Anything to be comfortable?
Not really—
There is a price to be paid: pain!

See if you recognize yourself on the following pages as you look at various sitting postures. Note the muscles that are involved, and the pain that can follow. Changes and stretches are suggested to help eliminate your pain problems. It is a journey worth taking!

Notes

"SLOUCH & LOUNGE" POSTURE

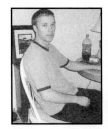 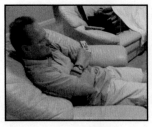 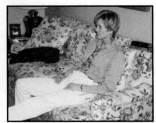

Yikes! Rounded back and shoulders, short abdominals, head forward, and tilted body. Those poor muscles are in such strained or crunched positions, they have to be uncomfortable when you stand up and unfold yourself. Rotate these pictures to see what these people would look like in a standing posture. If you stay sitting and lounging slouched long enough or frequently enough, it is difficult for the body to immediately become straight when you stand up, without eventually causing pain.

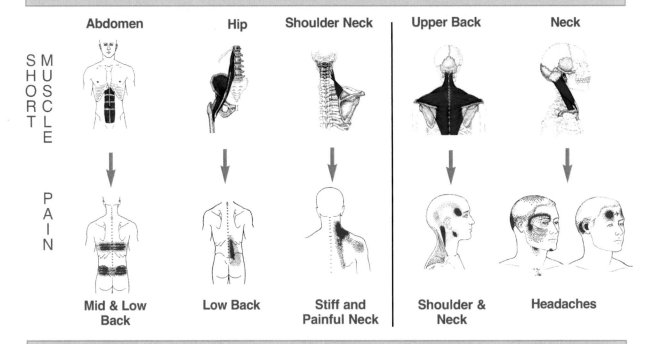

SHORT MUSCLE → PAIN

Abdomen	Hip	Shoulder Neck	Upper Back	Neck
Mid & Low Back	Low Back	Stiff and Painful Neck	Shoulder & Neck	Headaches

Not only can the slouch posture, whether sitting or lounging, give you pain, but it can affect your entire posture. Look at the postural changes in the photos below.

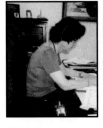 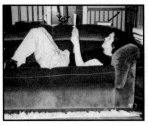 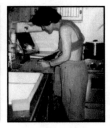 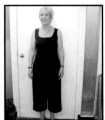

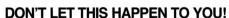

No back support and fatigued, the body slouches and the head is even more forward.

When relaxing at home, the head is propped forward, and the body crunched. This picture turned to a "standing position," shows you what her posture became.

DON'T LET THIS HAPPEN TO YOU!

At 48, she COULD NOT stand upright. She taught her muscles this posture and the spine followed forward.

TODAY! With postural changes and lots of stretching, she is upright again.

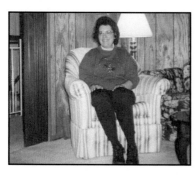
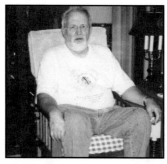
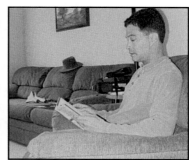

Corrected "Slouch" Posture

"Okay, okay. I get it. But how can I remember to always sit up straight when I just want to sit and relax? Besides, my furniture is so soft, I just sink into it."

Here are suggestions for making the necessary changes from the "slouch and lounge" posture:

Colored dots to the rescue
Place sticky, colored dots around the house and office, on the television, computer, telephone, and steering wheel, as well as in the kitchen, bedroom, and family room. The dot will remind you to check how you are sitting.

● ● ● ●

Pick furniture that allows good sitting posture
You should be able to sit with your buttocks to the back of the chair, sofa, or car seat. The back rest should be in a vertical position. If the back slants backwards, so will you. Then you tend to slide forward or to be in the slouch position. To help hold you upright, you may need a pillow behind your back (from the waist up, not behind your buttocks.

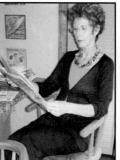
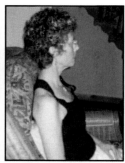

Be willing to try the new position
Avoid slouching or propping yourself up with pillows which leave you in a half-sitting, half-lying-down, slouched position. You really can be comfortable sitting up, and can eliminate the pain that comes from the slouched position.

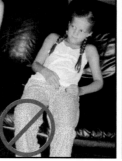
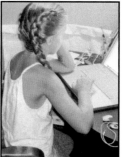

Incorporate stretching while you learn these new *habits*, and you will have a combination that is a true winner for ending your pain.

Stretching: a catalyst to recovery from chronic pain

Stretching = puts you in control of eliminating chronic aches and pains.
Stretching = allows you to be active, improving health and longevity.
Stretching = becomes a part of every day, reducing stress and leaving you more relaxed at the end of the day.
Stretching = if done correctly and frequently, initiates automatic comfort in movement.
Stretching = opens avenues for new activity, adventures, and experiences.

Wouldn't it be nice to have choices about what you do on your time off?
■ Be able to sit comfortably and in a way that will not eventually result in pain.
■ Have the energy to join friends for dinner, a game, or a movie.
■ Go for a walk without being fatigued and sore afterwards.
■ Take your kids for a day's outing without stiffness and achiness the next day.
■ Plan a vacation that involves hiking, beach walking, or scuba diving.

The list can be long, and you get to decide what's on it.

Wow! It sounds like stretching could be a good thing. But do I really have time for it? Yes. Follow "The Rule of Two" when doing the stretches suggested:

2 – Repetitions of each exercise presented, in the order they are given.
2 – Breaths are held on each repetition. This tells the body to relax, and that all is well.
2 – Hours before repeating the stretches.
2 – Sides of the body, not just the painful side.

This may sound daunting during a busy day. But you can find two or three minutes here or there. if you feel you can't, you're too busy.

Life is way too short to give up feeling good.

Stretches for reversing the muscle tightness resulting from sitting *slouched*

Stretching – You get to choose your own level of comfort
- Choose postural changes to reduce muscle strain.
- Choose postural changes and stretching, and you teach new *muscle habits* that allow freedom from pain when you are active. You can once again choose what you want to do, knowing your muscles are ready.

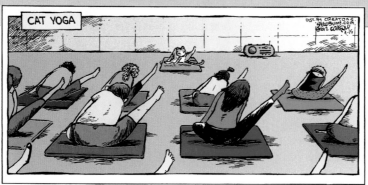

Speed Bump® copyright Dave Coverly/Dist. by Creators Syndicate, Inc.

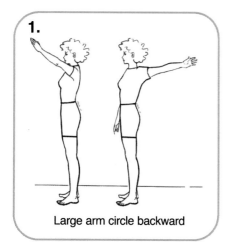

1. Large arm circle backward

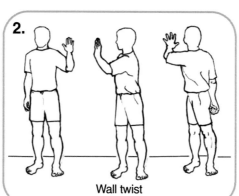

2. Wall twist

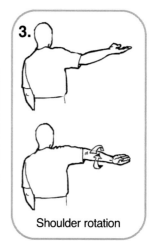

3. Shoulder rotation

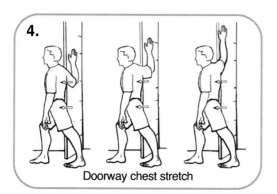

4. Doorway chest stretch

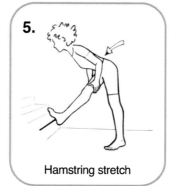

5. Hamstring stretch

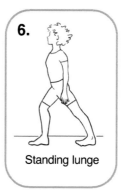

6. Standing lunge

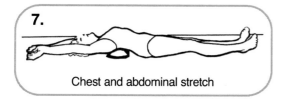

7. Chest and abdominal stretch

Please refer to **Appendix 1: Stretch Instructions** in the back of this book for more details on these stretches.

"PROPPED UP" POSTURE

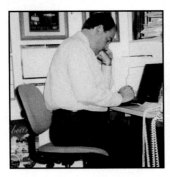
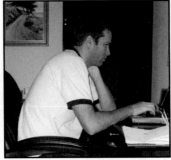
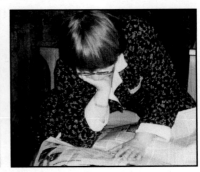

Oh! Just a little help, please.

"I am too tired to sit up straight, or maybe too involved in what I am doing, or the furniture isn't a good fit. Whatever!" The problem is that the bending-forward posture scrunches muscles in the front of the body that translate into back pain. The head is strained as well since it is positioned out in front of the body. Note below the muscles that are being misused and the pain that follows.

To sit leaning forward, with the head propped up in front of the body, the muscles holding that posture are strained. *Muscle strain leads to fatigue and pain.*

When you sit bent forward, crunching the muscles in front of the body, you find it takes a few minutes to stand up straight. Trying to stretch upward, lengthening the muscles, you experience mid- and low-back pain. Notice below that back pain is referred from muscles in the front of the body, not from the back. *Everyone thinks something is wrong with the back, when short muscles in front can lead to your back pain.*

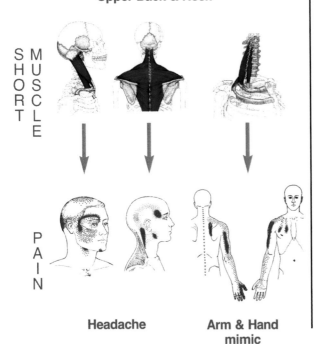

Upper Back & Neck

S H O R T   M U S C L E

P A I N

Headache   **Arm & Hand mimic "Carpal Tunnel Syndrome"**

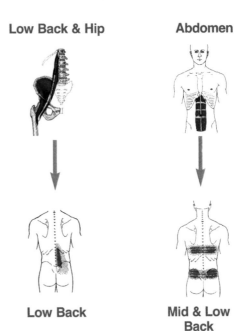

Low Back & Hip   **Abdomen**

Low Back   **Mid & Low Back**

68

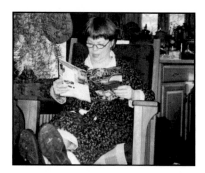 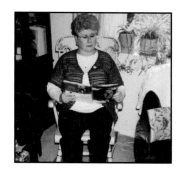

Corrected "Propped Up" Posture

"How can I remember to sit back in the chair
when I am comfortable and fully focused on the task at hand?"

Remember "comfortable" does not necessarily mean correct.
Taking a position that keeps muscles short, reinforces their staying short.
Short muscles usually result in pain.
Tension in muscles can only build up so long before the muscles can't function properly and pain results. If tightness continues, the pain continues and can become chronic.

Old sitting habits result in too much tension in the muscles and lead to pain.
Stretching, along with changing to new sitting habits, results in muscle lengthening and eliminates pain.

Suggestions that make a difference:

Colored dots to the rescue
Place sticky-colored dots ● ● ● ●
around the house and office: on the desk computer, telephone, television, and at the kitchen table or bar. The dots will remind you to check how you are sitting.

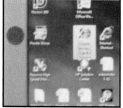 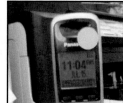

Choose the right chair
Find a chair that has only a slight backward lean, allowing you to sit with good back support. If necessary, use a wedge pillow behind you to help hold you upright.

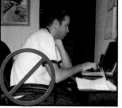 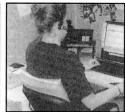

Take a break
Muscle fatigue often results in the body slumping and leaning forward. Take a break: take a walk, get a good snack or something to drink, or get together with friends. Then return to work.

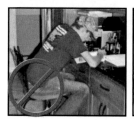 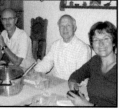

Stretch

Yes, you always put tension in and shorten your muscles as you use them. That is exactly why you need to sit correctly and stretch frequently. This prevents the muscles from being vulnerable to fatigue, cramping, injury, and chronic pain.

Stretching: easy but critical

"Why do I need to stretch when I've just been sitting around most of the time?"

Muscles are made to move. You can't get away from it. Muscles allow you to do everything you do. If muscles are allowed to get tight from not moving, they resist movement when called into action, which can result in achiness and pain.

Bones or muscles = pain? You often hear "oh, my aching bones." Although bones can cause pain, it has been my experience that the pain you feel is often is the result of tight muscles from too much sitting. Sitting may be your choice, or it may be a demand of work. Whatever the reason, you need to allow yourself opportunities to move throughout the day and in the evening.

> Muscles kept without regular movement and poor positioning result in muscle shortening and strain leading to pain. Stretching allows muscle movement with no pain.

Have you ever tried to see how long you can sit absolutely still? It is tough; your body wants to move. How much you sit, what posture you sit in, and what you do while sitting determine which muscles are strained and cause your pain.

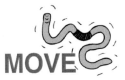

MOVE

Regular stretching, every two hours, needs only to take 1-2 minutes. Your muscles will be ready for more use, without fatigue, strain, or pain.

Follow these simple "Rule of Two" guidelines for stretching:

2 – **Repetitions:** do two repetitions in the order the stretches are listed. You do not need to do more.

2 – **Breaths:** take two deep breaths, then release the stretch (this lets the body know the stretch is a good thing).

2 – **Hours:** repeat the stretches every two hours. This helps teach the muscles to stay in this new position, rather than returning to old patterns of tightness.

2 – **Sides:** stretch both right and left sides, but separately.

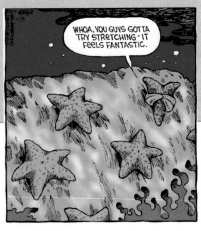

WHOA, YOU GUYS GOTTA TRY STRETCHING - IT FEELS FANTASTIC.

You will find nothing easier than 2 minutes of stretching to make you feel good, both physically and mentally.

Go For It.

"Speed Bump" copyright
Dave Coverly/Dist.
by Creators Syndicate, Inc.

70

Stretches for reversing the muscle tightness resulting from *propped-up* sitting

F O C U S

- **This** is a feel-good stretch, not a see-how-far-you-can-pull-the-muscle.
- **Feel** a slight stretch, avoiding a hard pull.
- **Hold** the stretch gently. It should feel good.
- **Avoid** bouncing with the stretch.
- **Everything** should be relaxed as you stretch.

1.

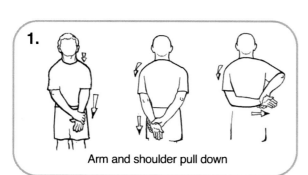

Arm and shoulder pull down

2.

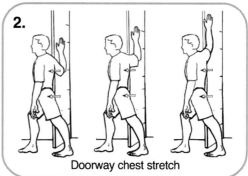

Doorway chest stretch

3.

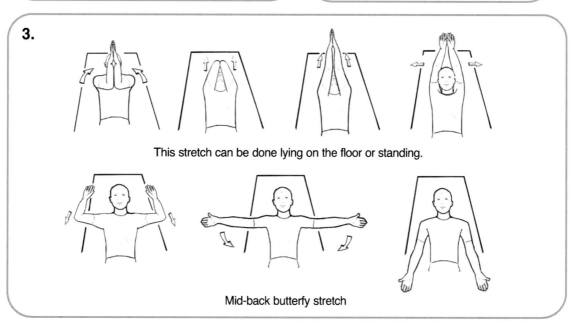

This stretch can be done lying on the floor or standing.

Mid-back butterfy stretch

4.

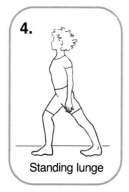

Standing lunge

5.

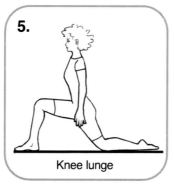

Knee lunge

6.

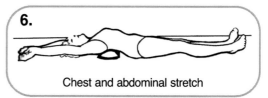

Chest and abdominal stretch

You Can Do It.

Please refer to *Appendix 1: Stretch Instructions* in the back of this book for more details on these stretches.

"TORQUED" POSTURE

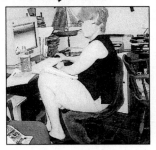 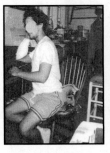 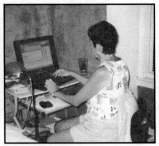 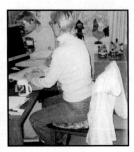

Ow! Sitting in this posture doesn't even *look* all that comfortable.
No wonder you hurt. Here's what happens:

Too often you sit torqued because of the furniture: the television only fits in the corner, and the desk you use really isn't a computer desk. Your knees don't fit under the desk, so you can't pull the chair close enough, or you need to arrange the monitor off to the side a bit. The sofa is such a great place to spread the paper and it seems okay to sit twisted to read it. If various situations did not dictate it, you would not stand or sit torqued because you would immediately feel the strain. Sometimes we just do things without thinking.

Take a look at the pain that can result.

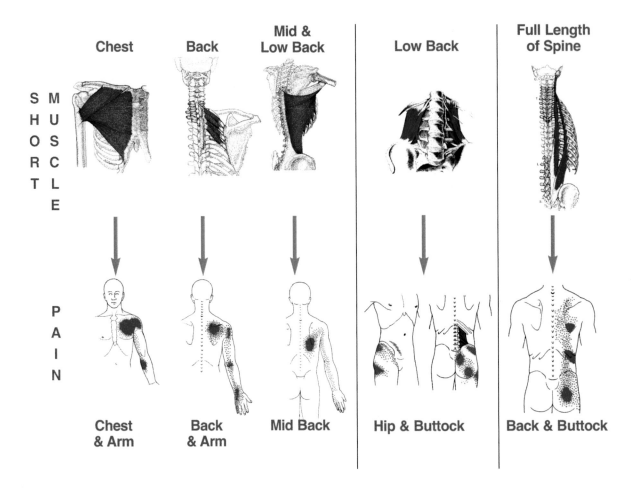

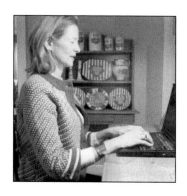
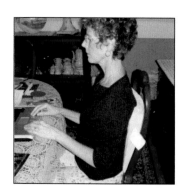

Make changes that allow your body to be straight. When you torque for only a few minutes, you think it is "no big deal." But it is: it keeps the body out of balance, which leads to pain.

Corrected "'Torqued'" Posture

Making changes isn't always easy. Here are a few hints to help:

New arrangements
Arrange furniture, computers, television, and games so they are directly in your line of vision, not off at an angle.

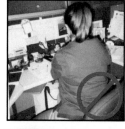
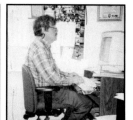

Choose the right chair, desk, or table
Find furniture that is high enough to allow you to pull your chair up with your knees under the table or desk.

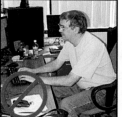
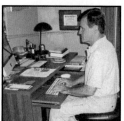

Choose to practice correct sitting
Once you make the decision to sit upright and facing your work, it will become an easy posture to take.

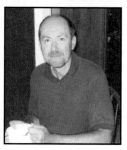

Stretch frequently
Frequency will help develop new *muscle habits,* making the new posture comfortable.

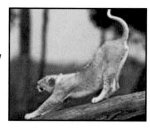

Yes, you may have to think through your furniture placement and maybe switch some furniture pieces with those in another room. It is worth it if it helps eliminate your aches and pains. To further aid you in achieving pain-free living, learn and perform the simple stretches on the following pages.

Ah, stretch!

Stretching, if done correctly, feels good and does not involve or result in pain.

> **Your muscles take a big sigh of relief as they relax and are allowed to repair and prepare for more movement.**

What is so important about stretches that you can't miss a day or two?

- Stretches release tightness in the muscles that accumulates throughout the day.
- Stretches move the muscles to a relaxed, resting position, allowing a return to full use. Stretching to full use teaches muscles new patterns of function that are not possible with tight muscles.
- Stretches establish *new muscle memory.* Muscles learn to do what you have repeatedly done.
- *Stretch memory* movements then become *muscle habits.* Remember, if you do anything often enough, it will become a habit. The same is true of *muscle movement.*
- New, elongated *muscle habits* help eliminate the stiffness, achiness, and pain caused by tight muscles.

You use your muscles all day long, in every posture and for every movement you make. If you do not stretch a couple of minutes several times a day, the tension has nowhere to go. Tightness accumulates or builds up in your muscles. This can lead to stiffness and achiness. Eventually, the tightness in the muscles builds until it results in pain. The pain can initially be occasional, and of varying intensity. At some point, if you do not stretch to eliminate the tightness, the pain becomes constant and begins to change how you live.

> **Take a break from what you are doing and stretch.**
> **It really does feel good, and it is good for you!**

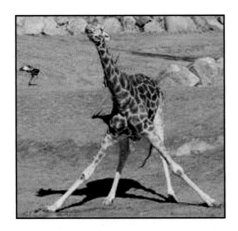

Stretches for reversing the muscle tightness resulting from sitting *torqued*

RULE OF TWO:

2 – Repetitions of each exercise
2 – Hours before repeating stretches
2 – Breaths before releasing the stretch
2 – Sides of the body to be stretched, one side at a time

Focus:

- **This** is a *feel good* stretch, not a *see-how-far-you-can-pull* the stretch.
- **Feel** a slight stretch, avoiding a hard pull.
- **Hold** the stretch gently.
- **Avoid** bouncing with the stretch.
- **Relax** your body as much as possible when stretching.

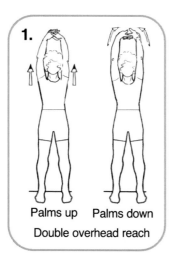

1.

Palms up   Palms down

Double overhead reach

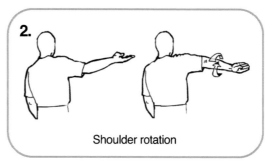

2.

Shoulder rotation

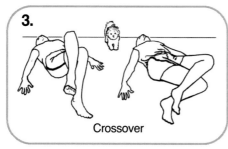

3.

Crossover

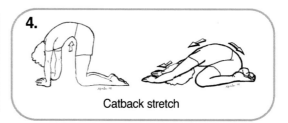

4.

Catback stretch

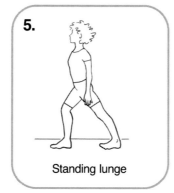

5.

Standing lunge

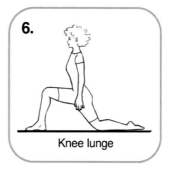

6.

Knee lunge

Stretches undo muscle tightness and release tension.

Please refer to *Appendix 1: Stretch Instructions* in the back of this book for more details on these stretches.

"SIDE LEAN" POSTURE

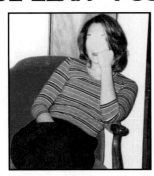

Notice as the body leans to the side, the head tilts the opposite direction to keep you balanced. This often triggers additional pain.

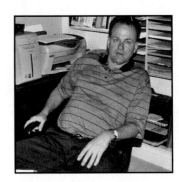

Auck! Why do you lean? It can be difficult to get comfortable. You may be trying to find a satisfying position, or the chair just isn't made to fit you. There are times you may lean without even thinking about it. The leaning posture shortens muscles that can result in pain, as shown below:

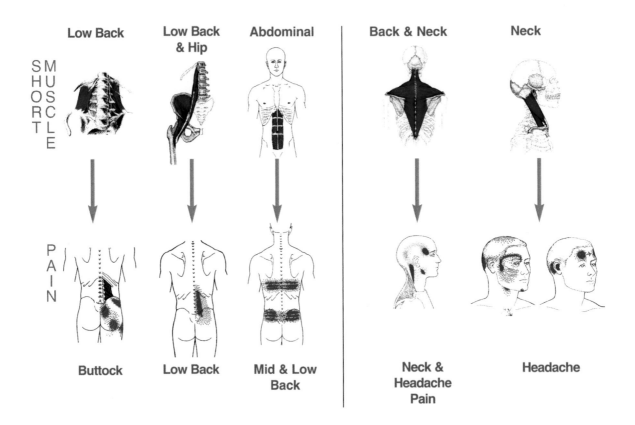

	Low Back	Low Back & Hip	Abdominal		Back & Neck	Neck
SHORT MUSCLE						
PAIN	Buttock	Low Back	Mid & Low Back		Neck & Headache Pain	Headache

Using a new sitting position and teaching your muscles a new, balanced position will greatly reduce the pain patterns above.

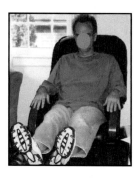

"I know I lean, but I just need to be comfortable. How do I do that without getting back into more pain?"

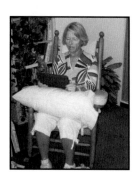

Corrected "Side Lean" Posture

Establishing new *muscle habits* will result in sitting comfortably without muscle stress. The postures shown above, coupled with the stretches on the following pages, will be instrumental in eliminating your pain.

You need to be in control of changing your pain. Don't let furniture have that control. Here are some suggestions to help:

1

Colored dots once again
Placed the colored dots around the house where you sit the most. They will remind you to sit more upright.

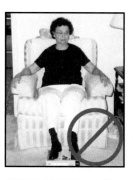
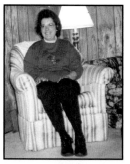

2

Choose furniture that fits you
The shape or contour of furniture can be too big or too small, not allowing you to sit relaxed, without muscle tension.

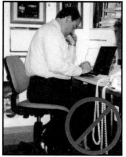
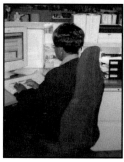

3

Leaning may indicate a difference in size on the right and left sides
Correcting the difference will allow you to sit evenly and relieve muscle stress.

Follow the principles and *specific stretches* on the following pages to develop new muscle habits that eliminate pain.

Stretching should not be a foreign word in your dictionary

It's common to think of stretching as a time-consuming, wasted-energy exercise? Many people are looking for strength and cardio workouts, so stretching may be limited to a few minutes before and after exercise, but not much more. You may have been taught that strength is more important than stretch. What is the issue?

Why, when, and how you stretch is crucial. When you are living with daily aches and pains, the rules change. Let's take a look:

Why?
■ Muscles need both flexibility and strength. Strengthening tightens muscles, and the shortness remains even when the muscle is at rest. Stretching returns the muscle to an elongated and relaxed position. The balance of strengthening and stretching keeps the muscles free of unwanted tension, decreasing the vulnerability to injury.
■ Stretching allows for greater strength. A muscle contracts for power. If a muscle is short, it has less capability to contract. A long muscle has more contraction available, so it is stronger.

How?
■ A stretch should be gentle, with a slight pull. There should be no bouncing movement.

How Long?
■ Hold the stretch while you take 2 deep breaths, allowing the entire body to accept the new muscle posture. Stretching to teach new relaxing *muscle habits* requires frequency, not long periods of time.

When?
■ Every 2 hours. Many people recognize they have tight muscles but do little to eliminate that tightness. Only when pain becomes an issue do they begin to take notice. To reverse the tightness, stretch often enough that the muscles learn *new patterns, new ways to work.* You can build the stretches into things you do every day: stretch when you step out of your car, get up from your chair, or wait in a shopping line or at a stop light. Stretches do not have to be cumbersome, just frequent.

Results?
■ Stretching establishes *new habits,* and as with all habits, stretches are best learned by frequent repetitions. Stretching only once a day for 20—30 minutes soon allows your muscles to return to their old, tight, pain-producing position for the rest of the day. Frequent stretching refreshes the muscles as you work, so you enjoy freedom from fatigue and pain.

■ Taking time off from work or an activity to rest a painful muscle is not effective. As you rest, you have not changed the *muscle memory* or taught the muscles to function differently. When you begin using the muscles again, they will function just as they did before. Stretching changes how the muscles work and therefore affects pain.

Stretches for reversing the muscle tightness resulting from sitting in a *side lean* posture

Okay, you are on your way, making postural changes, taking time to relax, and eating better, and you have already noticed aches and pains diminishing. Now for the last piece of the *feel-good* puzzle – stretching!

Apply The Rule of 2 and you continue to eliminate your chronic aches and pains.

Rule of Two: **2** – Complete two repetitions of each stretch. Remember these are to be gentle stretches, not pushing as far as you can.
2 – Hold each stretch for two breaths before releasing. Relax as you do the stretch, increasing the movement slightly as you exhale.
2 – Repeat each series of stretches every two hours. Remember, it is the frequency that teaches the muscles to stay longer.
2 – It is important to stretch both sides of the body, but separately.

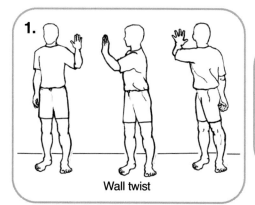

1.

Wall twist

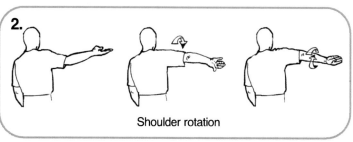

2.

Shoulder rotation

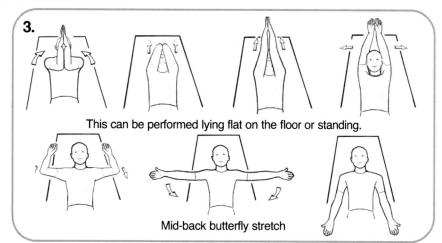

3.

This can be performed lying flat on the floor or standing.

Mid-back butterfly stretch

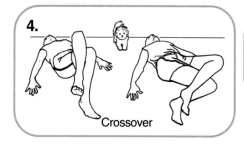

4.

Crossover

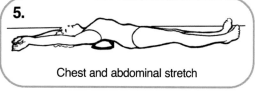

5.

Chest and abdominal stretch

Please refer to **Appendix 1: Stretch Instructions** in the back of this book for more details on these stretches.

"SIDE TUCK" POSTURE

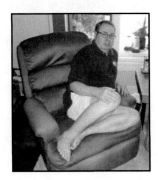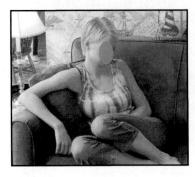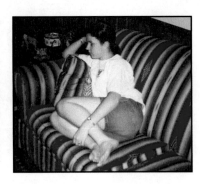

Oh! This "side tuck" posture looks like the knees and hips could really be stiff and painful when you stand up. Let's take a look at why:

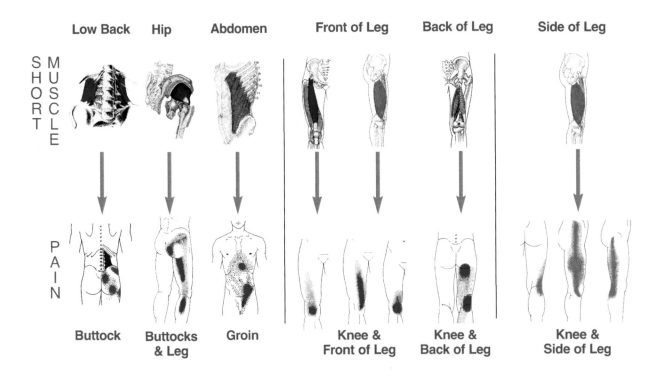

| Low Back | Hip | Abdomen | Front of Leg | Back of Leg | Side of Leg |

SHORT MUSCLE → PAIN

| Buttock | Buttocks & Leg | Groin | Knee & Front of Leg | Knee & Back of Leg | Knee & Side of Leg |

"Comfortable" carries so many meanings. When the body is out of balance due to short muscles, this "tucked" position is comfortable. Remember though, that "comfortable" in this case means an *adaptive* posture that will eventually results in pain. Unfortunately, it also creates pain when you stand up straighter to begin moving. There are ways to counter this tuck on the following pages.
No tuck = no pain!

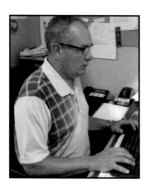

"It really is hard to change old habits, especially when I am so comfortable already. How do I make the change without going crazy?"

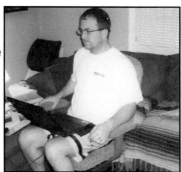

**Corrected
"Side Tuck" Posture**

Muscle tightness, left unchanged, will eventually result in pain! It isn't easy to make changes. Sometimes you aren't even sure you want to change. It takes time, energy, and focus to make real changes. But if it is the difference between being in pain and not having that nagging, chronic achiness all the time, it is worth it. You will be amazed that the changes aren't as difficult as you might think.

Pain unchecked means pain controls what, when, and how you do things.
Making changes to reduce pain puts *you in control* of what, when, and how you do things.

Hints for establishing a new sitting posture:

1

Colored dots to the rescue ● ○ ● ●
Place colored dots on soft and cushiony pieces of furniture that invite you to sit and to curl up with a good book or movie. Pick a different place to sit.

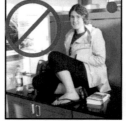
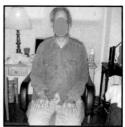

2

Choose furniture that isn't oversized, so there's no room to tuck your legs
Soft sofas and large chairs or recliners make it easy to tuck your legs off to the side. Select a chair that *fits* you, and sit with your feet on the floor or foot stool.

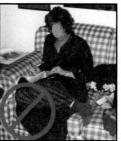
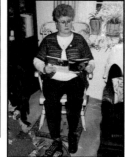

3

Check Chapter 4 to see if one side of your body is smaller than the other
Correcting differences between the right and left sides of your body makes it comfortable to sit evenly.

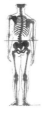

Come on, let's hear it for stretching!

What is the big deal with "stretch?"
Stretch is the key element in movement.

You all know what it is like to be tight: having a headache or a "crick" in your neck, having trouble getting out of a chair, avoiding stairs, having difficulty getting comfortable in bed, and being really careful so your back doesn't "go out."

You know you feel better when you do stretch: the knees don't crunch as much, you can reach up high to get things, you can put either arm in your jacket first, and you can reach around to tuck your shirt in or bend over to tie your shoes. You can take a walk or a jog up the street, or join in a family game of football or catch. Stretching lets things happen!

Stretching is as important, if not more so, than strength training. Strength comes from stretching. You won't develop strength if you are too tight to use your muscles at full capacity. Tight muscles are weaker than stretched, loose muscles performing at full capacity and full strength.

Just as you know you need to eat well AND get good sleep to be healthy, you need to stretch AND exercise to be healthy.

The Rule of Two for Stretching

2 — **Repetitions:** Complete two repetitions of each stretch.
2 — **Breaths:** Hold each stretch for two breaths before releasing.
2 — **Hours:** Repeat each stretch every two hours to develop *new muscle memory.*
2 — **Sides:** Stretch both sides of the body, but just one side at a time, to gain balance throughout the body.

Suggestions to help your stretch *feel good*

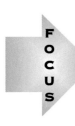

FOCUS

- This is a *get-rid-of-pain-stretch, not a see-how-far-you-can-push* stretch.
- You should feel a slight stretch, avoiding a hard pull.
- Hold the stretch position gently, without bouncing.
- Breathe normally throughout the stretch. The temptation is to hold your breath.
- Relax your entire body as much as possible when stretching.

Start and end your day with stretching!

Stretches for reversing the muscle tightness resulting from sitting with the *legs tucked*

1.
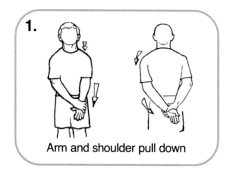
Arm and shoulder pull down

2.
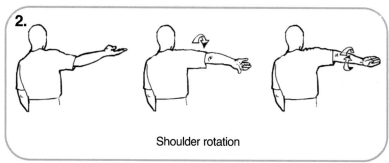
Shoulder rotation

3.
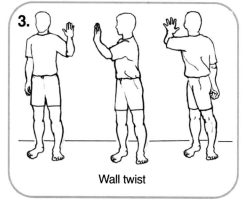
Wall twist

4.
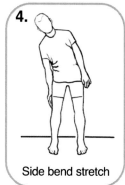
Side bend stretch

5.
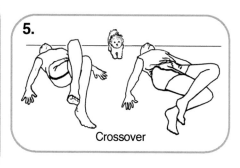
Crossover

6.
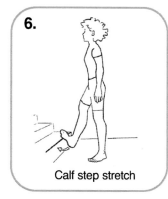
Calf step stretch

7.
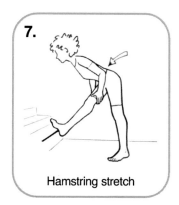
Hamstring stretch

8.
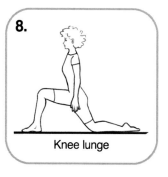
Knee lunge

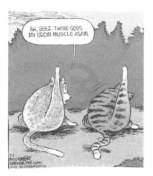

You are in control. Stretch away your pain.

Please refer to *Appendix 1: Stretch Instructions* in the back of this book for more details on these stretches.

"CROSS-LEGGED" POSTURE

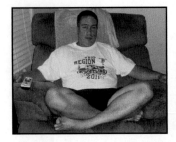 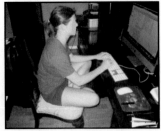 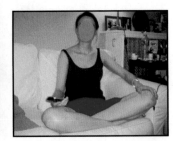

Ow! Those knees aren't liking this posture. Plus, look at the slouched position that goes with the crossed legs. A backache and even headaches can result.

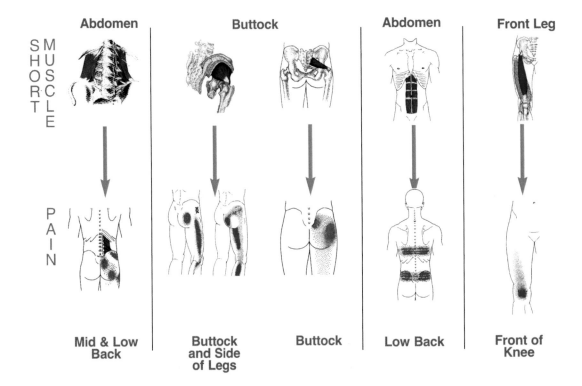

Abdomen	Buttock		Abdomen	Front Leg
Mid & Low Back	Buttock and Side of Legs	Buttock	Low Back	Front of Knee

(Left column labeled vertically: SHORT MUSCLE → PAIN)

You may sit cross-legged for a number of reasons: to meditate, to get your legs out of the way as you reach forward to do a task, to obtain a wider lap to act as a work surface, or just out of habit. Have you ever heard the saying "criss-cross applesauce"? This saying is often used with children to get them to sit quietly with their legs crossed and their hands folded in their laps. It is obviously somewhat comfortable, or people wouldn't do it. But remember, *comfortable* isn't always healthy in the long run. The legs are certainly in a strained position at the hips and knees. In addition to the pain patterns mentioned above, it is not unusual for the legs to cramp after sitting in this position. Muscles need to be in an elongated position to be free of tension when resting.

Muscles staying tight can result in pain, cramping, and even numbness.
Muscles long and relaxed result in pain-free movement.

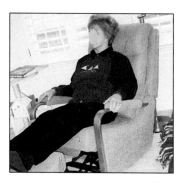 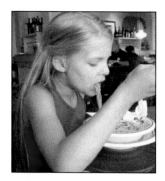 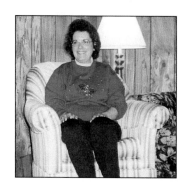

Corrected "Cross-Legged" Posture

Your Choice!

Untangle your legs and give the muscles a chance to be in a relaxed and ready position for whatever you want to do = no pain.

Keep the old habit of crossing your legs, and they will eventually cramp, tingle, and limit the activities you are able to do = pain.

Think about it. Is it really that difficult to untangle your legs and sit with them down? You can do whatever you decide to do.

"Okay, but how do I change the position when it is so hard to get comfortable?"

Here are a few suggestions to help:

Pick a chair or work area that gives you good support and alignment. You will experience less fatigue, achiness, and weakness. Plus, you will have more energy with your neutral sitting position.

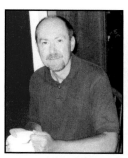 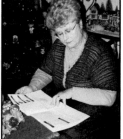

Choose to sit with your legs down in a non-strained position. Sitting with your legs out in front of you with your feet on the floor or on a foot stool.

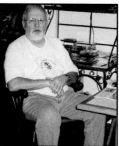 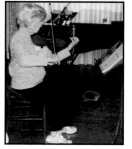

Stretch
You need to reduce the existing muscle tension to allow for movement without pain.

> **Let stretching help return muscles to good function.**

Good muscle use requires stretching frequently

Normal, daily muscle use increases muscle tension, and without stretching, tension builds, resulting in pain.

It is important to realize *why* pain happens so frequently. At some point, something has to empty or reverse the shortness in the muscles. They can only function with so much tension before they are vulnerable to cramping, strains, sprains, tears, and other injuries. The buildup of tightness doesn't happen in an instant; it can be the result of a cumulative buildup over days, weeks, and months.

Normal, daily muscle use interspersed with stretching releases muscle tension and eliminates pain.

As stretch intervenes throughout the day, muscle tension is removed, eliminating a buildup of tightness and tension and avoiding painful results.

Stretching can be as easy as 2-2-2-2!

2 – Repetitions: You don't need a lot of repetitions when you stretch frequently. Good *muscle habits* are established with you repeat the same movements often, rather than a lot of repetitions just once or twice.

2 – Deep Breaths: Hold each stretch for 2 deep breaths to let the brain and body know this movement is good. This will enhance the relaxation of the muscles. Sometimes you don't even have a lot of time to hold the muscle stretch. Not to worry: short duration with frequency does the job.

2 – Sides of Body: While you may have pain or tightness on only one side of the body, it is important to stretch both sides. This maintains a good balance in the muscles for optimal use.

2 – Hours: Stretch every 2 hours. Remember, it is the frequency of teaching the muscles what you want that establishes what they will do.

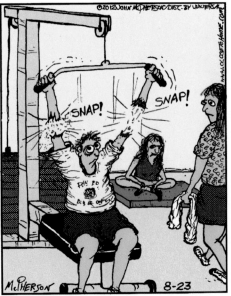

Tim forgot the importance of stretching out before hitting the weight machine.

Everyone has time for the above protocol — everyone. How long does it take to do a few stretches just 2 times? What about doing them while waiting for the elevator, in a meeting room, in the grocery line, waiting at school to pick up your child, listening to the news, or during commercials on TV? You deserve to feel good. Stretch to change your life.

Stretches to reverse the muscle tightness resulting from sitting in the *cross-legged* posture

I know you are busy. There is always something or someone making demands. There just isn't enough time.

I understand. That is why this program is made simple and quick. Check it out! Remember, it will only take 2—3 minutes. You deserve at least that much time to be healthy.

Do the stretches in the order listed.
The floor stretches can wait until you get home.

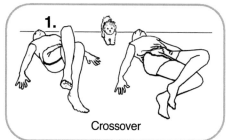

1. Crossover

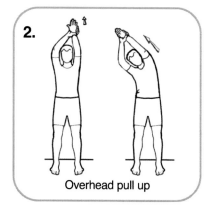

2. Overhead pull up

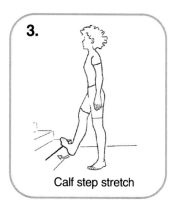

3. Calf step stretch

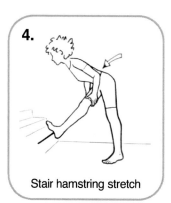

4. Stair hamstring stretch

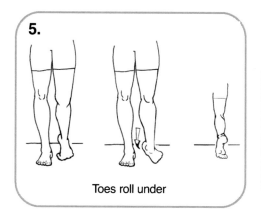

5. Toes roll under

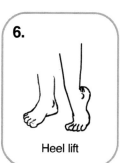

6. Heel lift

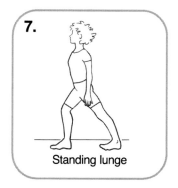

7. Standing lunge

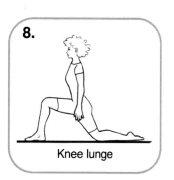

8. Knee lunge

Please refer to *Appendix 1: Stretch Instructions* in the back of this book for more details on these stretches.

CHAIR SUMMARY

What do chairs really have to do with sitting?

Ouch! Most chairs, stools, loungers, recliners, sofas, and other sitting furniture are not comfortable: too small, too big, too soft, too hard, no backs, curvy backs, slanted backs, scooped seats, tilting seats, seats too short or too deep.

Very few pieces of furniture are designed for comfort and proper sitting. Consider the following:

Recliners – Reclining invites you to take the slouch sitting posture.

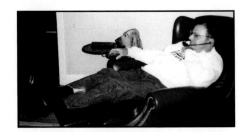

The headrest usually pushes the head and shoulders forward.

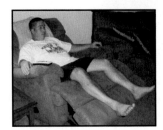 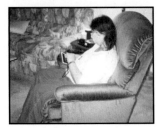

Slanted-Back Chairs – Without a high, straight back for support, you often take the *propped up* or *forward lean* posture with a back rounding and the head jutting forward.

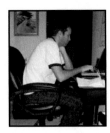 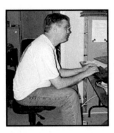 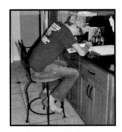 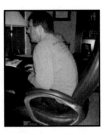

Zero-Gravity or Wavy Chairs – These chair backs keep you in a curved *slouched* position, similar to the recliner. Unlike the recliner, however, the seat slants at a significant angle backward, moving the pelvis into a backward tilt and jammig the hips.

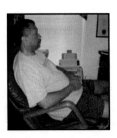 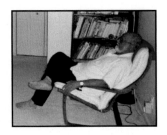

Casual or Dining Chairs – Chairs for more casual sitting are often made to fit no one in particular. It is most common to find the depth of the chair seat too long. If you were to sit all the way back in the chair, your feet would not reach the floor. Pillow props or "lean" positions are often the result of trying to find comfort.

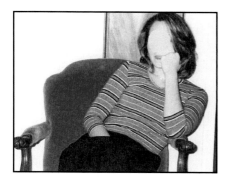 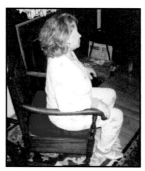 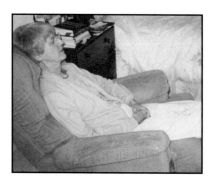

It is easy to find yourself using chairs that are not comfortable. Your chairs may be family hand-me-downs or you found them before a great sale price, or the colors match the rest of the room. Maybe you merged two homes and you got what you got.

Just as mattresses are a major factor in good sleep, so chairs are a critical part of sitting comfortably. Once you begin to change your posture to fit your chair and begin squirming around to get comfortable, you are changing your muscle's habits that will take you down the road to achiness, followed by more serious pain.

Pick chairs for comfort, not just looks.

Decide on the function of the room and the chair before buying.

Chairs need to fit. Sit in one and try it out before you buy!

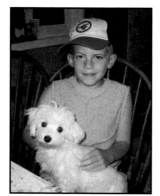 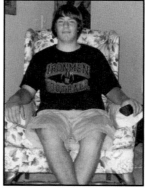

Good sitting

CAR POSTURE

The same principles apply to sitting in cars as to sitting on furniture

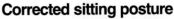
Corrected sitting posture

■ **Center of hips, shoulder, and ear in a straight alignment**
Keep the seat back in an upright position rather than leaning backward. This avoids the head jutting forward.

Head forward = headache and stiff neck

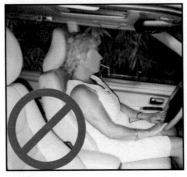 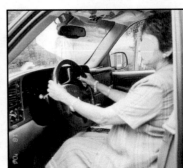

■ **Curved space behind the back filled in with a wedge pillow**
Curved seat backs allow you to sink into a rounded back and crunched posture in the front of the body.

Body rounded = mid- & low-back and hip pain

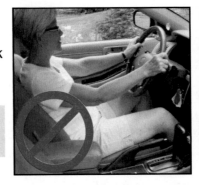 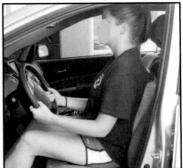

■ **Headrest should not push the head forward**
Forward headrest pushes the head out in front of the body, straining the neck and upper back.

Head forward = headache, stiff neck, and shoulder blade pain

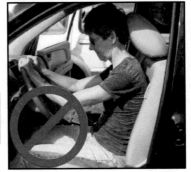 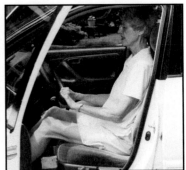

■ **Car seat should be level front to back and side to side**
A backward-slanted seat causes a tight bend at the hips. Side edges slanting upward can cause you to sit lopsided.

Too much bend = low back pain
Uneven side to side = hip pain and leg pain, mimicking "sciatica"

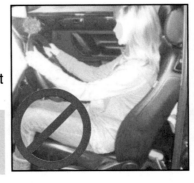 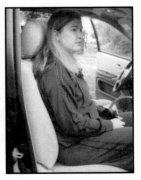

Making these simple changes can make driving comfortable, even enjoyable!

Notes

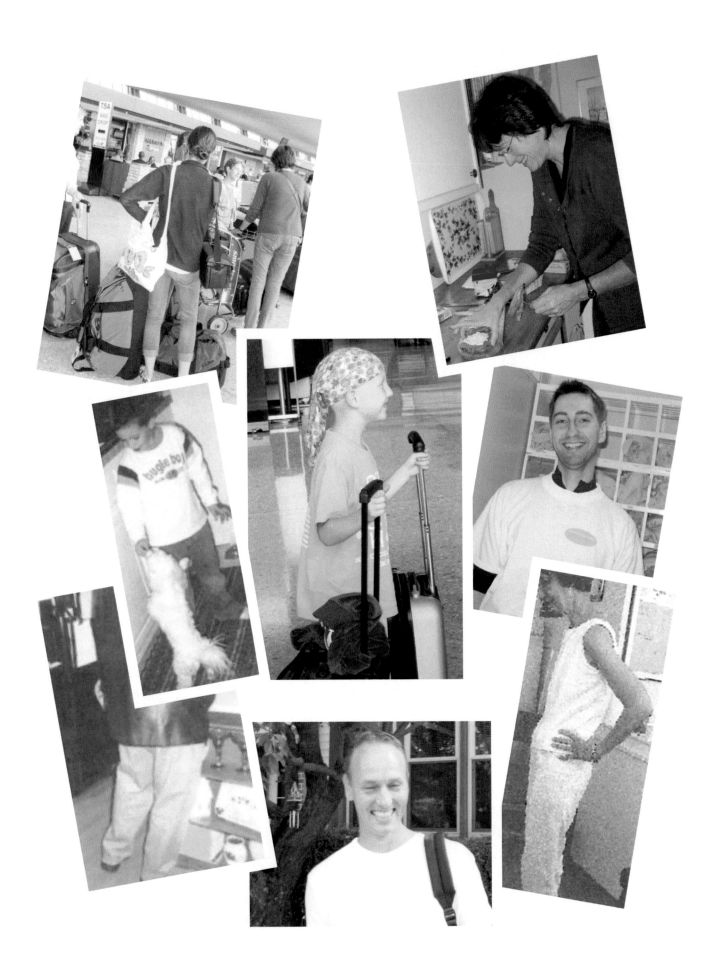

Chapter 4.
Standing: Not Always an Easy Thing to Do

*W*hen you watch people stand around talking, notice that most of them do not really seem relaxed and comfortable. They move around, shift their weight, lean against something, twist and turn the shoulders, or just squirm. If you ask them about it, they often respond that it is so much easier to walk around than to just stand still. Why is that?

The following are conversations with patients as they sought treatment for pain associated with standing.

Ann. "Hi. I'm just calling to see if you deal with pain that I feel mainly when I stand. I can stand for only a few minutes before my hip pain is so intense I have to sit down, and sitting is just about as bad. Is this something you treat?" Ann asked when she called the clinic.

"Yes," I assured Ann. "I work a little differently than most therapists, but this is definitely something I can help you with. It is common for treatment to address where you have the pain, but I look at *how* your muscles are functioning and *why* using them is resulting in your pain."

To help unravel this pain mystery, I scheduled a consultation with Ann and asked that she bring photographs for review of her muscle use: sleeping postures, watching television, cooking, vacuuming and cleaning around the house, working at the computer at home and work, positions in the car, doing yard work, and anything else she does as hobbies or activities.

"Do I really need pictures?" she asked. "I can show you all of the postures and whatever else you want when I come in."

"That won't be effective," I said. "We need to look at your postures as you cook, clean, sit on your chairs and sofa, and lie in bed—and whatever else you do throughout the day. You'll see that the pictures will help identify the stressed muscles that are part of *why* you have pain."

When Ann arrived for her appointment, she sat across from me and before long, began to squirm. After squirming for a while, she tried standing. I could see why she was uncomfortable. She was leaning to the left when she was sitting and had the same tilt when she was standing. I asked Ann if she was leaning because of pain or just trying to get comfortable.

"I didn't realize I was leaning," she said, "but it isn't because I hurt. I guess I just seem to lean that way. When I stand, it seems that I'm always shifting from one foot to the other, kicking one leg out to the side or trying to lean against something for support. When my back and hip pain get worse, I try different positions, even if they help just a little."

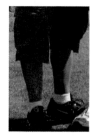

As an experienced pain therapist, I recognized that Ann's back and hip pain could be caused at least in part by what is called a *leg length inequality*. The difference in the right and left sides of the body is a common factor in perpetuating chronic muscle pain. Let's take a closer look at what this involves.

It is important to understand that leg length inequality is not necessarily an actual difference in the length of the leg bones. You move because of soft tissue that is attached to bones. Soft tissue is the combination of muscles, tendons, ligaments, cartilage, and connective tissue. Any difference in the combination of these soft tissue factors on the right and left sides of the body results in a leg length discrepancy. With so many soft tissue components involved, it is easy to see how a leg length difference could arise.

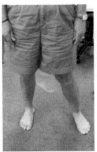

To further verify the difference in her leg length, I asked, "Ann, have you ever noticed a difference in shoe size, one foot smaller than the other? Or a difference in ring size between your right and left hands? Many people are structurally smaller on one side than the other. Many people are aware of such differences, but not to the extent of realizing they can be a part of chronic pain. You already mentioned standing with one leg out to the side or in front of you. Have you also noticed one pants leg hanging longer or your dresses hanging unevenly?"

"Oh, yes," Ann said. "All those things. In fact, some therapists have told me I have one leg longer than the other, but the amount is so little that it doesn't matter. Others say it is so minimal they can fix it with adjustments, but it always seems that my clothes are crooked anyway. If it really is such a small difference, can it be that important?"

I explained that even if the unevenness in your hip and leg is as little as one-quarter inch, it could be a difference of over one inch at the shoulder level. Think of a seesaw. It may be level to begin with, perfectly balanced, but if you move the center point even a small amount, one end will go way up in the air.

Based on years of looking at leg length differences, I told Ann I was certain she had a leg length imbalance, and it could be one of the causes of her hip pain. She seemed puzzled with that comment. "I was concerned at first because some therapists told me my legs were uneven, so I had them X-rayed. The doctor told me the bones were exactly the same length. Plus, I have had several treatments when I have been checked before the session, and I was uneven. When I was checked after the treatment, I was even. So, how can one leg be longer than the other? This isn't making sense."

"Ann, it sounds as though you were lying down when you were evaluated for this leg length difference, but has anyone ever checked you while you're standing?" I asked.

"No," she said. "You're right. I've always been lying down for an X-ray or on the therapist's table. Why? Does that matter?"

I explained that we are not talking about structure, the actual length of the bones, when we evaluate a difference in leg length. We are talking about function. Bones don't move by themselves; they move because muscles are attached to them. Other types of soft tissue such as ligaments, joint cartilage, and connective tissue hold bones together, cushion joints, and allow movement. When the muscles move, the bones move. If you X-ray bones or check leg length only when a patient is lying down, soft tissue is not working, so you're evaluating bone length from the X-ray. Because bones alone don't determine leg length differences, evaluating function correctly requires observing the way all the types of soft tissue are working in a weight-bearing situation. That is why it is so critical to check for leg length difference from a standing position: when you are standing, your body engages all those wonderful bone and soft tissue parts so you can balance and remain upright. That is when we need to evaluate leg length—while you're using your legs.

Here's an example. Let's say you want to choose a door for your home. You have two pictures: one shows an ornate door with beautiful carvings, and the other shows a door that is chipped and needs to be painted. Your choice, of course, is the beautiful, ornately carved door. What you can't tell from the pictures is that the ornate door has rusty hinges that don't work, while the paint-chipped door has new, well-oiled hinges that work perfectly. Static pictures are not helpful in evaluating the door's function, but if you open the door, you engage all of its parts. Once you open the door, it is easy to check for a problem, fix it, and return the door to its full function. The same is true when evaluating leg length differences. A static view of a patient lying down doesn't show all the factors involved in movement. Thorough evaluation for leg length discrepancy must be done while the patient is in function; that is, standing.

I wanted to move on to the pictures Ann brought to see if they showed some of the same possible issues I had already observed in the office. "So," I said, "let's take a look at your pictures to see if there are other indications of a tilting of the body to one side." I wanted Ann to study the pictures with me, so she could understand how imbalances could be a factor in her pain.

As we went over the pictures, Ann noticed that in the photos where she was standing—

- Her pants leg was definitely longer on the left side. "That means I'm short or smaller on that side, doesn't it?"
- Her left hip was lower than her right, causing her waistband to slant down to the left.
- Her left arm hung away from her body, while her right arm hung against her side.
- Her left shoulder was higher than her right. "Why is my left shoulder higher than the right shoulder and my shirt moves off to the right, if I'm smaller on the left side? Shouldn't the left shoulder be lower, just like the left hip?"

"Think about it," I said. "You are smaller on the left side, which causes you to tilt in that direction. Your body tries to compensate by bringing the left shoulder higher than the right to balance with the low left hip. With the left shoulder high, your shirt will shift to the right. The body is basically trying to keep your eyes level. If both the hip and shoulder were low, you would be walking around bent over sideways. Your body is quite clever at compensating to keep you even."

After looking at the pictures, Ann and I talked about a few additional steps to document a leg length difference. You can follow these same steps to see if you also might have a leg length imbalance that could be part of your chronic aches and pains:

1. Stand barefoot in front of a mirror in non-baggy clothes. See if *one arm hangs further from the body* than the other arm does, or if your arms hang evenly against your body. The arm on the body's low side generally hangs further from the body if you are tilted to that side.

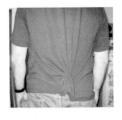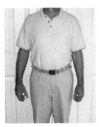

2. Look at your sides. Is *one side straighter* than the other, without much of a curve in the "love-handle" area? The higher hip has more of a curve. The lower side tends to be straighter, as the muscles are pulled longer in order to attach to the top of the low hip.

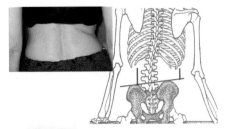

3. Look at the length of a pair of pants you are wearing. Does one pants leg hang longer than the other? The short leg is the one with the pants hanging longer, as the body leans in that direction.

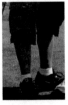

4. Stand barefoot and place your feet a few inches apart. Put your arms out in front of you at shoulder height. Have someone press down on your arms while you resist (don't let them push your arms down). It is not a contest, so don't go crazy making it one.

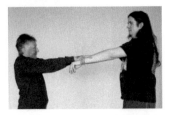

5. Do your arms drop easily or *can you hold the straight arm position, firmly resisting the push?* If the arms drop easily, this is another indication that you have a leg length difference. You are weaker because you are uneven. It is like standing on the side of a hill: you are not as strong or as balanced as when you are standing on level ground.

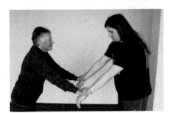

6. Have someone sit in a chair behind you while you are seated and use their index fingers to *feel for the top of the hip bones at the sides*. From the position of the fingers, you can see if one side is lower than the other.

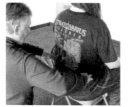

7. Does your shirt slide down your shoulder to one side? It is common to see the shirt slide to the side opposite the shorter leg. Remember the shorter, or smaller, leg side is the high-shoulder side, as the body seeks to obtain evenness and balance. One shoulder low and one shoulder high are indications of leg length inequality.

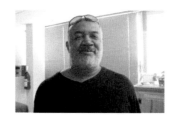

8. Have someone watch you walk. Do they notice a *slight limp* or *rocking* as you walk? You rock from the long leg to the short leg, landing harder on the low side. This gives you a side-to-side *rocking* look as you walk. The stress of landing harder on the short side with every step can be a factor in giving you hip pain on the low side.

Any "yes" answers on these simple tests usually indicate a muscle imbalance from a leg length difference. Knowing this can give you a better understanding of why you have chronic pain. The differences may be subtle or more dramatic. Remember though, a difference of only *one-quarter inch* can become a major factor in how muscles function. If the right and left sides work differently, one side generally gets more stress, which can result in hip, low-back, and leg pain.

Once Ann saw that she had a leg length discrepancy, her next question was quite logical. "So what do I do about this leg length thing so I can get rid of my pain?"

I explained I would put a heel lift of one-quarter inch in the heel of the shoe of the short leg. "The lift raises the short side of your body to the level of the other side, allowing more even, balanced movement. If your shoe has an insole, we can put the lift under it to help hold the lift in place. A heel lift will need to be placed in every shoe or slipper you wear, so there is a consistency in the muscle lift positioning. No going barefoot; barefoot puts the muscles back in an uneven position from right to left since there is a leg length difference. It becomes difficult

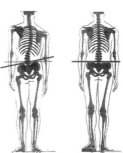

Without lift   With lift

for the muscles to learn to function in the new position with the lift if you sometimes use it and sometimes don't. Muscles that are consistently even with the lift will develop new habits of functioning from a balanced position. Your hips will be even, and there will be no leg length difference, allowing the muscles to function without pain."

"I assume you'll give me a lift today," said Ann, "but what happens when I need more lifts for other shoes?"

"You may be able to find heel lifts on the Internet or at a local store." (A list of suppliers for the recommended heel lifts is found in the *Contact and Products Resources* appendix.) "But," I cautioned Ann, "there are several considerations to keep in mind when you shop for the lifts."

- The lift needs to maintain the one-quarter inch height throughout the heel area before it begins to taper. A consistent one-quarter inch correction over the entire heel surface levels the entire body.

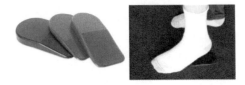

- Too many lifts on the market taper immediately from the back of the heel forward, a design that does not give full correction. When a lift tapers immediately, the correction for balance is lost.

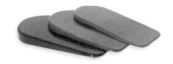

- It is critical to select a lift that is solid rubber or a compressed material, such as cork, to give a firm and steady correction. Many commercial lifts are made of soft, cushioning material that is not effective for lifting support. They may be a useful cushion for people having other issues such as heel pain, but soft heel lifts do not serve to provide the needed lift under the short leg needed to balance the body.

- On the other hand, it is not necessary to buy a hard plastic or custom orthotic when you are simply trying to add the quarter-inch at the heel level. Although custom orthotics are helpful for a number of foot issues, this is not one of them.

Share this information with friends and family. Anyone who follows the simple steps for evaluation and determines he or she has a leg length discrepancy can make a temporary lift for use until a "real" lift can be obtained. The temporary lift can be made in the following way:

- Fold a standard paper towel until you have a piece about 2 inches wide, 4-1/2 inches long, and 3/8 inch thick. It will compress down to about one-quarter inch as you wear it.

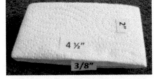

- Place the folded towel in the heel of the shoe on the side determined to be the low side. You may need to cut the corners so the folded towel fits into the back of the shoe.

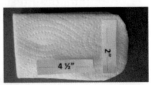

- Be sure the thickness is the same throughout the heel area.

- Try the arms-extended resistance test you did earlier. You should be able to easily hold your arms out in front of you once the lift is in place.

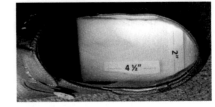

I find that a one-quarter inch lift is right for most people, though some will need less and some more. You can fine-tune the amount that's right for you by doing the arms-extended resistance test with slightly different heights under your heel. You might start by standing with 120 pages of a paperback book or magazine under your heel. Then try a few pages less each time, until you find the correct thickness needed to allow you to hold your arms strong and steady on the arm resistance test.

"Oh, I'm sure some of my friends must have this same leg length problem," said Ann. "So why don't they have the same pain I do?"

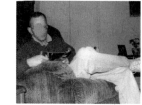

I explained, "Not everyone who has a leg length difference experiences pain." People frequently accommodate a leg length discrepancy by crossing their legs when sitting or kicking a leg out to the side when standing. These corrections work temporarily, since those accommodations provide balance for a leg length difference while decreasing stress on the affected muscles and joints. Remember, though, when they start walking or driving a car, they can no longer cross the legs or kick one leg out to the side. Without these adaptations, the leg length discrepancy can cause muscle stress and fatigue, and eventually can be a major factor in hip, back, and leg pain. If someone's work allows them to sit, only occasionally getting up to move around, the leg length issue may not be a problem for some time. It is also important to remember that muscle pain comes from a combination of perpetuating or contributing factors.

"The combination is different for every individual, which means that the pain results will also vary from person to person." I further stressed that it is not wise to compare one's pain with that of others. Think about people who wear eyeglasses. The prescription they need, and when they need to wear their glasses or don't, varies with each person. Likewise, your pain is unique. But if it's needed, using a heel lift will prevent muscle imbalance from becoming a pain problem.

Ann was excited that something as simple as identifying and correcting the leg length difference eliminated her hip and back pain. Now that her body is balanced, she can stretch to help keep her muscles loose and ready for new adventures.

> **Never forget**
> **that real healing**
> **begins from within:**
> **Accepting, then implementing**
> **changes that will bring about**
> **pain-free living!**

Judy. Judy is at a great place in her life. She retired from a desk job earlier in the year and has been enjoying her free time working on new lawn projects. But Judy has been finding it harder to stand comfortably after all the bending, squatting, and kneeling in her new rock gardens. Her knees have become so sore she is finding it hard to enjoy the coed softball games she began playing with other retired friends. A former patient, she called me at the clinic. "Hey, you fixed my back a while ago, and I was wondering how you are with knees."

I told Judy that muscles can also be the culprit in knee pain, and we needed to take a look at what might be causing the problem. I reminded her to bring in new pictures to evaluate her muscles while sleeping, watching television, working at the computer, working around the house, doing the lawn projects, and even playing softball. "Judy, how about bringing a few pairs of shoes with you, too? Casual, as well as the ones you wear for gardening work and for playing softball."

"Shoes I can do, but pictures may not be so easy," Judy responded.

"Judy, the information we'll get from your new pictures will be as valuable for fixing your knees as your earlier pictures were for figuring out your back problem. If we can't see what you do with your muscles, it is difficult to figure out what started, and what is perpetuating, the pain."

"Got it," she said. "Can I bring the pictures in my camera, or do they have to be printed out?"

"On the camera is fine," I replied. "I can put your camera card right in my computer, and we'll take a look."

It is common to evaluate pain by going directly to the pain site—in this case, the knees—and checking leg strength and stability. My approach with Judy was to be quite different. Because there seemed to be no specific incident that caused the pain, but rather a change in activities, my focus would be on function instead of structure. After discussing her new activities, we began to talk about what factors could be contributing to her knee pain. Judy hadn't really thought about what positions she used while working in the yard, but she was able to figure out better work habits without much help. She just needed to focus a bit on taking nonstressful postures: lifting without twisting, and moving closer to the objects she was lifting rather than reaching and lifting.

Looking at other contributing factors, we corrected her leg length difference, as we had done with Ann. Then we moved on to other issues, ones not commonly addressed. Judy brought out several pairs of shoes she wore for working in the yard and for playing softball. Shoe structure can cause foot and knee stress, as well as dictating how she walks. Her softball shoes were so stiff that a good bending motion was not possible. Without thinking about it, this caused Judy to change the way she walked and ran for several hours at a time at softball practices and games. She did what she had to do, accommodating the stiff shoes by running rather flat-footed and hiking her hips to move her leg forward. She realized it was shortly after she began playing ball that spring that her knee pain got worse.

On the other hand, her yard shoes were an old pair that she used as "mud shoes," but they were too wide and not very supportive. The poor fit and lack of support required a number of foot muscles to grip just to keep the shoes on and maintain balance. No wonder her knee pain got worse. Wearing shoes that were flexible and supported her feet was an easy solution for both softball and working outside. (See the chapter on shoes.)

Being out of balance had also changed Judy's standing posture. As Judy and I took a closer look at her standing posture, it seemed to me she was leaning backward. As I looked at her from the side, I could see that her shoulders were further back than her hips and her upper back was rounded. Judy felt as though she was standing straight and tall, lined up correctly with hip, shoulder, and ear in a straight line. She was unaware she was leaning backward. I then took a picture of her standing, from a side view. She found it hard to believe that her weight was shifted almost entirely to her heels, and it looked as though she had to really work at not falling over backward.

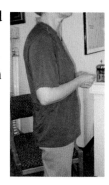

"That is interesting," said Judy. "Balance has become a real issue since I started playing softball. Fielding a ball, and even batting, throw me off balance."

As a therapist dealing with how people function, I was taught to listen to patients, and they would often tell me what issues were involved in their pain and movement problems. With Judy's mention of balance, we switched our focus to her center of gravity. If it was compromised, it would surely be part of the problem causing stress on Judy's knees.

By leaning her body weight backward, Judy forced the muscles in the front of her body to stay tight in order to hold her upright and keep her from falling backward. The pull of the front thigh muscles had a direct impact on Judy's knees. Muscles in the thigh attach across and around the knees. The pull from the tightness in these muscles was felt where they attached, which was at the knees. Muscles in the back of her legs also tensed to try to hold her upright. Pain behind the knees could result.

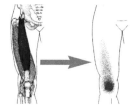

I asked Judy to shift her weight to the center and even forward toward the balls of her feet as she stood, and I took another picture. The second picture showed Judy with her weight shifted forward, off of her heels. Standing in this weight-forward position and without forcing the change, Judy brought her hip, shoulder, and ear into a straight line, in perfect alignment.

"This feels really weird." Judy laughed. "I feel like I'm going to fall over." After a few minutes she said, "Wow, I definitely feel better balanced. I can even feel my hip and leg muscles begin to relax. I can feel less pressure on my knees when my weight is more in the center and forward on my feet. I think I feel less strain on my back and neck too. Is that possible?"

"It sure is," I responded. "If you look at the first picture I took of you, with your weight back more on your heels, you can see that your mid back is overly rounded, your low back is flat, and your head reaches forward. Without the normal curves, your low-back muscles are pushed into a difficult work position that produces strain. Your head-forward position requires the mid- and upper-back muscles to tighten in order to hold your head. Changing your center of gravity by shifting your weight forward allows the normal curves to return to your back and neck, changes your balance, and positions your muscles to function efficiently and without strain. This can significantly reduce your pain."

Judy realized she would have to pay attention to how she stands. Her weight has been back on her heels for so long that the muscles have learned to work in that position. Judy's compromised posture, in this case leaning backward, is incorrect but fixable. "I'll probably have to ask my family and friends to give me a signal when I stand with my weight back, at least until I get it right," Judy offered thoughtfully, already on her way to healthier knees.

> **You do not need to see
> too far ahead.
> Just take the first step
> and let the changes follow.**

Henry. Henry, a high school student, was diagnosed with shoulder tendinitis and a partial frozen shoulder. His mother called to ask, "What exactly is tendinitis? Is that the same as a partial frozen shoulder? I have heard they are really the same thing. In any case, can you help with these kinds of problems?"

I explained that tendons are extensions of the muscle that attach muscles to bones. "If muscles get tight and pull on the tendon attachments at the joint, the tendons become irritated and inflamed. The term "-itis" at the end of a word means inflammation; therefore, tendinitis is inflammation of the muscle tendon. Henry's tendinitis is inflammation of some of the muscle tendons attaching at the shoulder joint.

"A *partial frozen shoulder*," I continued, "involves a group of muscles that have become so tight that they allow little shoulder movement, usually above shoulder height, without eliciting pain. If the shoulder is painful to move, it is easy for you to go ahead with many daily activities simply by bending at the elbow instead. You can do these movements without pain, so shoulder movement, itself, can become quite limited before you accept and seek help for the problem. A partial frozen shoulder indicates some movement restriction rather than a limitation of all movement at the shoulder, which would be called a frozen shoulder. "

"Medicine can treat the inflammation," I said, "but why is the inflammation there? Treating the inflammation alone, without eliminating its cause, is generally only a temporary solution."

I wanted to take a look at how Henry was using his muscles and what he was doing to cause them stress. If we could identify and change the things that were causing the inflammation and stiff shoulder, Henry could obtain permanent pain relief.

As with other patients, I asked Henry to bring pictures of himself sleeping, reading, studying, sitting at the computer, watching television, using electronic devices, and playing his favorite sports.

"I guess these pictures don't look so hot, do they?" Henry said as he handed me the pictures at our first appointment. Henry carried a big backpack on his shoulder as he walked into the office. When I asked about the backpack, he said that he carries it around during the day at school and then carries a sport duffel bag on his shoulder after school for his sports practices.

"Henry, throwing those backpack and duffel bag straps over just one of your shoulders causes a few problems:

- The weight causes compression on the shoulder muscles, and they contract in response.
- Since you carry one bag or the other virtually all day, the compressed and stressed muscles are learning to work in a shortened position.
- Your muscles become tight, overloaded, and strained.
- The pull of your muscles on their attachments at the joint has caused irritation and inflammation."

"Another problem," I continued, "is that you hike your shoulder to keep the backpack or the duffel bag from slipping or falling off."

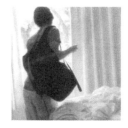

"It really doesn't feel so bad with the bags on my shoulder," he said. It's when I take them off and my shoulder drops down that I really feel the pain. What's up with that?"

"Let's look at what's involved:

- Hiking your shoulders means that every time you carry a bag on your shoulder, you are training the upper-back and shoulder muscles to be contracted, or short.
- The shoulder has to be hiked up so that your bags don't slip off.
- You've hiked the shoulders so much that the muscles have now learned to work from that shortened position. They have lost the muscle memory of functioning in a normal, shoulder-down position.
- When you try to lower your shoulder once the bag is removed, it's painful because you've lost your normal range of motion for those muscles. They only know how to function short or hiked up.
- The shoulder muscles hurt when you drop them down to a regular position, so instead of trying to position them down, you accommodate the muscles, finding ways to shorten them again: putting your hands on your hips or folding your arms across your chest, both of which raise the shoulders.
- That accommodation of keeping the shoulders lifted up, the continual shortening of the muscles, is not only painful but can eventually lead to a partially frozen shoulder."

Henry and I began looking at some of his other pictures. He said, "Look at that! My shoulders are rounded and my head is just hanging out in front of me when I have the bags on my shoulder. I guess you just sort of do that when you have bags up there. They are so heavy you lean and round the back to counterbalance the weight in back."

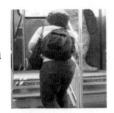

We talked about how the constant weight of a bag on his shoulder causes his muscles to fatigue and his shoulders to round, as he observed earlier. Rounded shoulders and the head forward can easily result in headaches, a problem he began noticing the week before.

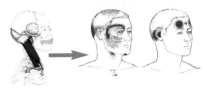

"Rounding your shoulders also places the muscles in the front and back of your shoulder into imbalanced positions and restricts shoulder movement. Some back muscles are pulled forward, while front muscles are contracted or bunched. This puts stress on both sets of muscles as you attempt arm and shoulder movements. This constant stress, of hiking the shoulder and the compression from the weight on your shoulders, is probably a big factor in your inflammation and partial frozen or stiff shoulder."

"I really need to fix this shoulder," Henry said with some urgency, "or I'm going to lose my place on the baseball team. Besides, a bunch of my friends and I are heading for the beach over spring break for some surfing, and shoulders are really important for that."

"Henry, let's start by using the backpack as intended, with a strap on each shoulder, which allows them to stay down. Better yet, skip the backpack for a couple of weeks and add some gentle shoulder stretching."

"The duffel bag has to come off the shoulder, too," I said. "Carry it in your hand, down at your side. That constant pressure on your shoulder muscles was too much and has caught up with you. The partial frozen shoulder is the result."

These changes will decrease the strain on the muscle and their attaching tendons, decreasing tendon irritation and allowing the inflammation to be treated successfully. Not carrying the bags on his shoulders for a couple of weeks would also give Henry time to work with stretches to teach the muscles to learn to function in their relaxed, normal, elongated position, helping to reverse his partially frozen shoulder.

Adding a solid stretching program will help teach Henry's muscles to regain full movement, so he can be ready for that surfing vacation.

> **First say to yourself what you would be; then do what you have to do!**
> —*Epictetus*

The challenge starts today—will you join in the journey to pain-free living?

Notes

"HEAD DOWN" POSTURE

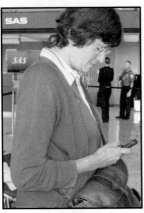
Texting

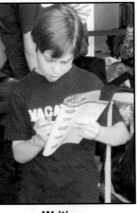
Writing

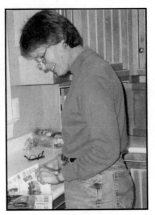
Reading

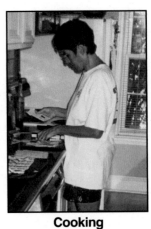
Cooking

Ouch! "My neck is so stiff. Pulling and pain start at the base of my head and go all the way down my back.

The headaches are dull, but they are there all the time. What is going on?"

Let's take a look at the head position for the answer.

Any time the head stays dropped down, the following strains are evident:
- Strain at the base of the neck
- A hard pull at the base of the head
- A pull that continues down the back between the shoulder blades
- A pull from the neck to the top of the shoulders
- A tightness in the muscles in the front of the neck

With the head at a significant downward angle, the muscles of the neck and upper back, indicated below, are in a strained position while holding the of your head. This muscle strain results in the pain shown here.

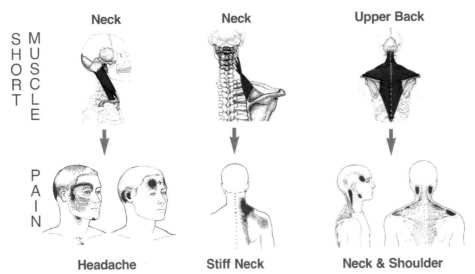

SHORT MUSCLE

Neck	Neck	Upper Back

PAIN

Headache	Stiff Neck	Neck & Shoulder

All of this pain, just from keeping the head down. You can feel the pull, may even rub your neck a bit, but too often you don't change the posture. You just keep doing what you are doing. The following page offers some simple solutions to help avoid this painful situation.

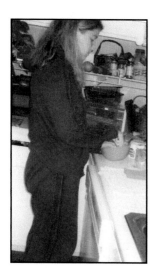

Standing too close to your work usually requires you to hold your head straight down to see what you are doing. Considering your head weighs 8—12 lbs, it is in your best interest to keep that weight more balanced over your spine and body. When the head is positioned forward, the strain begins at the base of the head and can go all the way to the low back. Moving back allows your head to be more upright.

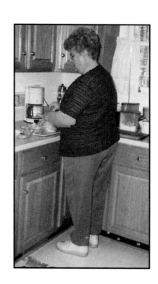

Corrected "Head Down" Posture

How does change happen? Simple suggestions are shown below.

Use a slanted surface
This brings the work to you rather than lowering the head in an extreme way.

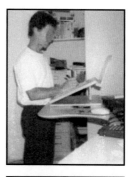

Why these suggestions work:

The head will be tilted down, but only a little.

Use an elevated surface
This brings the work to a level that allows you to maintain a more upright position without strain.

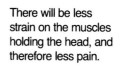

There will be less strain on the muscles holding the head, and therefore less pain.

The muscles shortened in the front of the neck return to a more lengthened position = less headache pain.

Bring devices to shoulder height
Avoid lowering the head to see the screen. Holding the device in front of you keeps the head more upright.

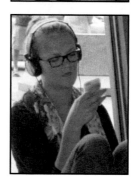

Once you get in the habit of standing this way, you will wonder why you didn't do it sooner.

Stretching

How can I convince you that changing a few postural habits and stretching are two of the most important things you can do to keep muscle health, and therefore yourself, healthy for a long time?

Constantly using electronic devices with the head down has created one of the newest "pain syndromes."

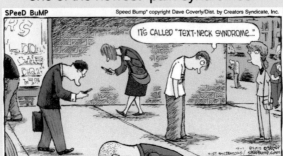

You often begin taking a slouched sitting posture that accommodates this habitual neck position

Chronic Pain

Think about all of the factors that invade your day that put tightness in your muscles, tightness that results in pain.

Stretching is one thing that relieves the shortness of muscles and allows them to lengthen, ready for you to use them without strain. Otherwise, tightness continues to build in the muscles until they respond with pain. Pain becomes chronic as muscles are allowed to stay tight instead of being stretched to a relaxed, non-strained position.

Stretching principles for chronic pain are different than stretching for flexibility. This protocol makes *feel good* stretching for pain reduction easy to accomplish:

- no specific equipment needed
- no specific place required
- no lengthy time requirement

Yep, just doing my neck rotation stretches!

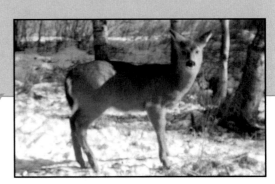

Stretches to reverse the muscle tightness resulting from the *head down* posture

The Rule of Two for Stretching

2 — Repetitions: Complete two repetitions of each stretch.
2 — Breaths: Hold each stretch for two breaths before releasing.
2 — Hours: Repeat each stretch every two hours to develop *new muscle memory.*
2 — Sides: Stretch both sides of the body, but just one side at a time, to gain balance throughout the body.

Focus: Suggestions to help stretch away neck and shoulder pain:·

- This is a *get-rid-of pain* stretch, not a *see how-far-you-can-push* stretch.
- You should feel a "slight stretch," avoiding a hard pull.
- Hold the stretch without bouncing.
- Breathe normally when stretching. The temptation is to hold your breath.
- Relax as much of the body as possible when stretching, including the muscles being stretched.

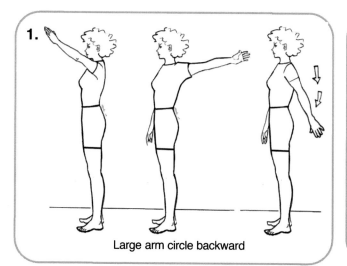

1. Large arm circle backward

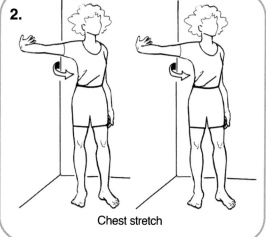

2. Chest stretch

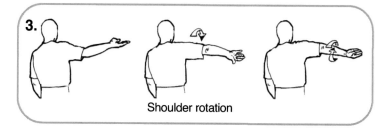

3. Shoulder rotation

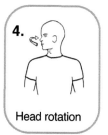

4. Head rotation

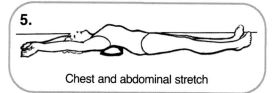

5. Chest and abdominal stretch

**Try it. It really works.
This can be the difference
between pain and freedom!**

Please refer to **Appendix 1: Stretch Instructions** in the back of this book for more details on these stretches.

"FORWARD BEND" POSTURE

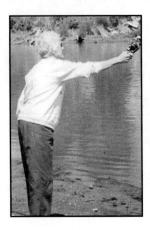 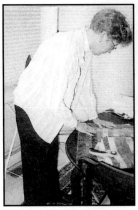 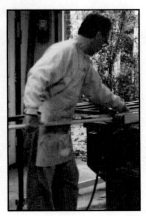 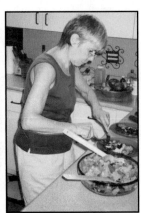

Yikes! You do a lot of different things during the day that don't really have you bending very much.

Besides, it doesn't feel bad at the time you're doing it. But just wait until later on, your back is killing you. Why? Let's take a look.

When you shorten the two muscles shown below by bending forward, even slightly, you have shortened the muscles that are responsible for the majority of all back pain. Yes, back pain can come from muscles in the front of the body, not from the back.

Short Abdominal Muscle   **Short Hip Muscle**

S H O R T   M U S C L E

P A I N

Mid & Low Back   **Low Back**

So much attention is given to the back itself when you have back pain. But almost 30 years ago, medical research published by Janet G. Travell, M.D. and David G. Simons, M.D. described the pain referral patterns that illustrated how back pain is "referred" from the tight muscles in front of the body shown here. Abdominal and hip muscles shorten from bending forward and elicit back pain.

Learning that back pain can primarily refer from short abdominal and hip muscles, it now makes sense that when treatment and rehabilitation, including stretches, are aimed at the back, pain persists. Tight abdominal and hip muscles in the front of the body shorten as you bend and lean forward with almost all daily activities and movements. Without adding stretching to counter this bending, it would make sense that these muscles can cause back pain. Stretch retraining and lengthening these muscles has given countless people lasting relief from their back pain.

Follow the suggestions offered on the following pages. The combination of the posture changes and stretching will work to give you a new freedom to move without pain.

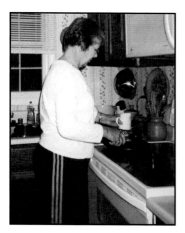

Obviously, there are times you have to bend forward, like getting into the trunk of your car. But there are times you can work in an upright position that allows the muscles in the front of the body to line up over your spine. This gives more support = less muscle strain and tightness. Tension from slightly bending forward, will build during the day, and by evening the muscles may be so tight you begin experiencing back pain. **Stand tall!**

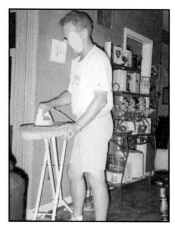

Corrected "Forward Bend" Posture

Standing seems pretty straightforward, yet slightly bending forward as you go about your day, is often the "why" behind your back pain. I can think of a number of things you do during the day that require bending forward. The challenge is to identify the times you do not have to bend forward, when you just do it out of habit. You can do many of your daily activities in a position that keeps you more upright. Remember, the majority of back pain results from *muscles in the front* of the body being short. Below are some suggestions that will help keep those muscles in a more neutral, relaxed position.

1

Make working surfaces fit your activity
If your working surface is too low, you have to bend to use it. Find a more suitable, higher place.

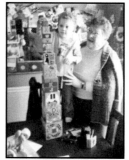
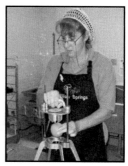

2

Use slanted surfaces when possible
A flat surface can cause you to bend your body forward and your head down. Using a slanted surface, or creating one for your book or project, allows you to stand upright and relieves tension in the neck as well.

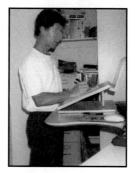

Don't let bending forward give you back pain.

3

Choose to stand upright when you can

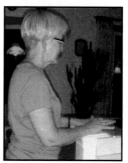
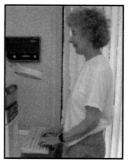

Stretching

Here we are again, talking about stretching. If you can grasp the value and importance of stretching, you will be in a position to turn off your pain. So much pain, especially chronic pain, comes from muscles, not from bones, disks, ligaments, or cartilage. Inflammation is real, but where does it come from? When muscles are allowed to get too tight, they begin to pull on their tendon attachments. If the tendons continue to pull, they get irritated and inflammation results in the entire area of the attachment. Unless you eliminate the tight muscle pull, the inflammation continues or returns even if treated with medication.

How do you get rid of the pull? Stretch! Stretch! Stretch!

All of the chronic pain we are talking about is from muscle dysfunction. There is nothing *wrong* with the muscles, they have just learned to *function incorrectly.* They have learned to function short. They are short because you use them every day, all day, without much, if any, stretching. Instead, you change the way you use your muscles, thus accomodating the shortness.

Stretching can be easy and takes only a couple of minutes throughout the day to be effective. **Yes**, you need to make the postural changes mentioned throughout the book. Those changes undo the accomodations you have used to be comfortable and to *keep going* throughout the day. The new postures release tension in the muscles and allow them to be ready for stretching. Stretching takes the muscles the next step, to working free of tension and pain.

The simplicity of stretching:
2 – repetitions, no more, no less. It is frequency that releases tension.
2 – sides, not just one side. Only one side may hurt or be tight, but to keep a balance in the body, stretch each side separately.
2 – breaths, no more, no less. It is not necessary to hold the stretches a long time.
2 – hours. Remember, it is the frequency you are after. That is what changes what muscles do.

Your Focus:
■ This should *feel good.* Don't *see how far you can push* the stretch.
■ When you first begin to feel a stretch or pull, stop and hold the position.
■ Hold the stretch steady, no bouncing. You want the muscle to learn to stay long.

**Stretching does not interrupt your life,
it gives it back**

Stretches for reversing the muscle tightness resulting from the *forward bend* posture

A little stretching = great results!

Do the stretches in the order they are listed, and remember "FOCUS" from previous page:

Please do your stretches frequently

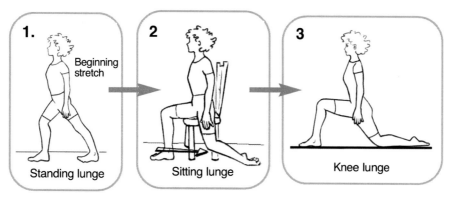

1. Beginning stretch — Standing lunge
2. Sitting lunge
3. Knee lunge

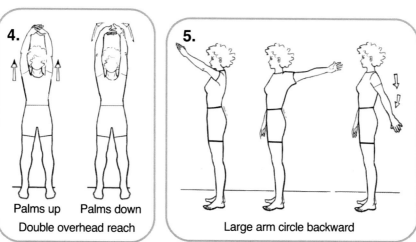

4. Palms up   Palms down — Double overhead reach
5. Large arm circle backward

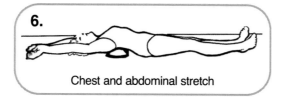

6. Chest and abdominal stretch

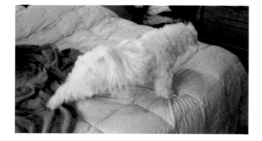

Easy breathing helps muscles relax to obtain maximum results.

Please refer to **Appendix 1: Stretch Instructions** in the back of this book for more details on these stretches.

"SHOULDER HIKE" POSTURE

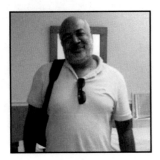 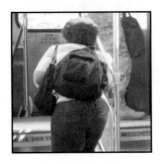 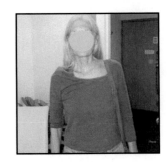

Ooe! "My neck and shoulders are killing me, and I am really starting to get a major headache."

How many times have you heard this statement?

When you carry a bag over your shoulder, it doesn't matter if it is light or really heavy. You have to *hike or lift* your shoulder to keep the strap from sliding down. With a bag over each shoulder (more common than you may think), you raise *both* shoulders to keep the straps in place. You eventually shorten and tighten neck and shoulder muscles to the point of producing pain.

Why do you do throw the bag on your shoulder?

■ It is easy and keeps your hands free.
■ It allows you to carry multiple bags easily.
■ It is such a habit, you just do it.

The most frequently affected muscles are shown below:

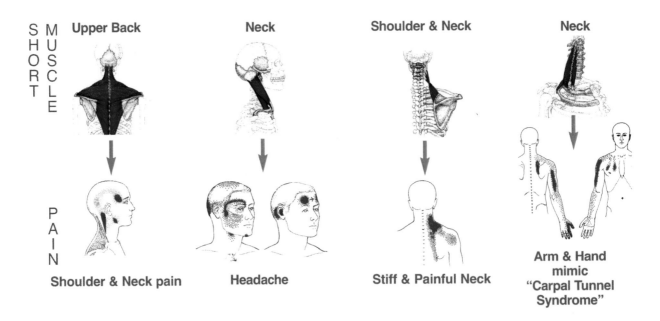

Besides pain, repeatedly lifting the shoulder commonly results in shoulder tendinitis, bursitis, and nerve impingement. Is it worth it?

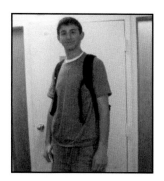 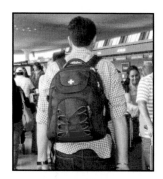 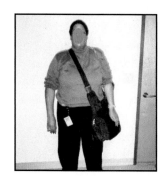

Corrected "Shoulder Hike" Posture

Most pain elimination does not come from a pill or happen in a doctor's office. Freedom from pain comes from identifying *why* you have pain, making informed changes that alter *old habits* of how you use your body, and establishing *new habits* that will allow your body to function without pain.

Changes are fairly simple for avoiding pain when carrying things:

- The obvious one is to use both straps for backpacks so the weight is evenly distributed.
- Use a backpack that is centered closer to your hips than your mid-back.
- Use a backpack, bag, or purse with wide or padded straps to distribute the weight on your shoulder.
- Decrease the weight in the bag.
- Use a roller bag.
- Put the strap over the head onto the other shoulder, where it can't slip off and still keeps your hands free.

Stretches for reversing the muscle tightness resulting from the *shoulder hike* posture

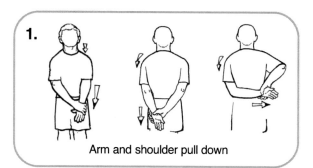

1.

Arm and shoulder pull down

THE RULE OF TWO APPLIES:
2 — Repetitions
2 — Breaths
2 — Hours
2 — Sides (both)

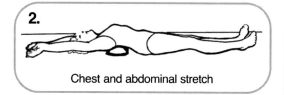

2.

Chest and abdominal stretch

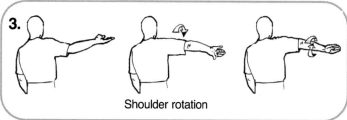

3.

Shoulder rotation

"SIDE LEAN" POSTURE

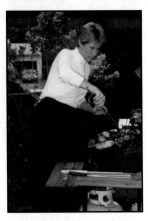 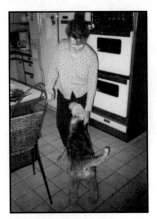 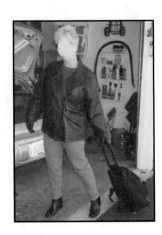

Oo! Leaning to the side looks like it might cramp your side.

Notice how the head tends to lean in the opposite direction from the body lean. Why do you lean when you don't have to? It is usually something you do out of habit, but it does cause some pain problems.

Leaning to the side shortens or bunches the side muscles shown below. They may not hurt at the time, but if you lean when sitting and standing, the shortness becomes too much for the muscles to handle. Back, hip, and groin pain can result.

Tilting the head in the opposite direction of the body lean shortens muscles that can lead to a stiff neck, headaches, and arm and hand pain and numbness that mimics *carpal tunnel syndrome.*

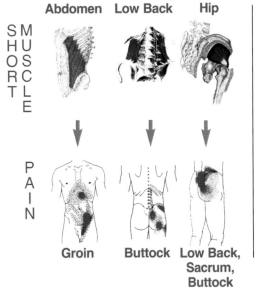

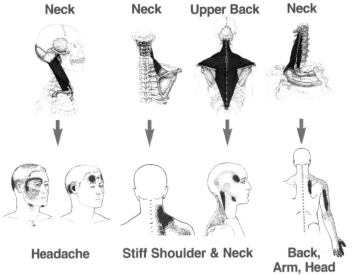

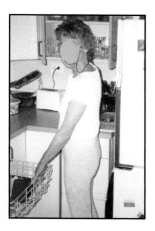

How do I change? It is just standing.
It is so easy to get yourself in a tilted or leaning position. But when you think about it, it is just as easy to stand straight. That is the key, think about it! You tend to rush around, keeping busy, not noticing your posture. Make a simple decision to notice and to stand tall in your stance. That one decision can go a long way in eliminating that chronic pain.

Corrected "Side Lean" Posture

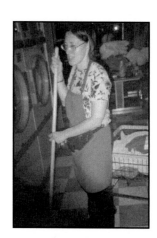

Standing straight can be easy if you become aware of how you stand. Because you have tightened your muscles during the day while sitting, and continue that shortening at night while sleeping, it is expected that those same muscles will take the same tightened positions when standing. Look at the progression of this man shown below to see how you can end up in a leaning posture from other postural miscues.

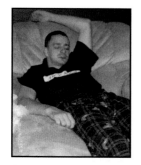
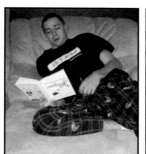
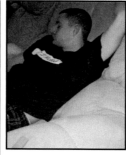

Sitting slouched and torqued.

When the pain increases, he tries a new position. He ends up like this.

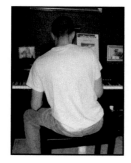
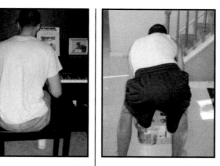
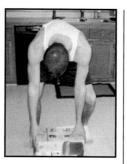
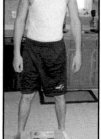

His sitting posture became the posture he used slouching. He feels like he is sitting straight.

Completely bent over. He says it is very strange looking at the pictures because he tries to bend straight and doesn't realize how badly he rotates. It has become muscle habit.

Side leaning and totally off balance; the lounging and sitting dictated his standing postures.

Since hip and back pain can come from the side leaning, take a moment to check what you are doing and make the effort to take an upright posture.

Awareness and choice are the key to standing tall. Stretching then teaches the muscles to function correctly.

117

Stretch

Stretching is the link between a sedentary lifestyle and pain-free health. I know, many jobs are sedentary. It becomes necessary for people in these jobs to get up frequently and move: take a walk, stretch, anything to loosen up.

What keeps people from stretching:

- People work out in the gym for strength training and cardio, feeling it is much more productive.
- Stretching doesn't feel like they are doing anything. There is no sweating, no gasping for air, no working for the *burn.*
- They do a few stretches here and there before they start their real workout.

Your ancestors, and perhaps even your parents, certainly lived a much more active lifestyle than you do. The advances of the machine age, and then the electronics age, allowed a great deal of work to be accomplished without much physical activity. But with those advances has come an epidemic of stress-filled lifestyles that result in chronic pain. What happened?

We have forgotten:

- Our bodies are a storehouse of leashed energy and pent-up stress if we do not release them through movement.
- Flexible muscles and free-flowing movements are great for stress release. There are few natural outlets for stress without movement. Without stretching, muscles become tight and weak.
- Stretching brings muscles to a suppleness or flexibility that allows easy, flowing movement.
- The muscles' being supple forms a bridge, a transition, from work inactivity to an active, energetic way of life.
- Stretching is as important as sleeping and eating in increasing stamina and movement capability; decreasing stiff, stressed muscles; and enhancing strength and wellness.

There is no substitute for stretching!

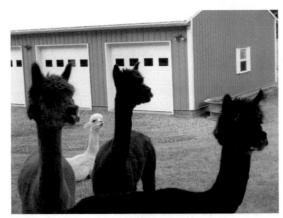

Let's stretch—All together now

Stretches for reversing the muscle tightness resulting from *side lean* posture

As stretching is built into your day, something you do regularly, you will begin to see freer movement, greater energy, and pain-free days. How good is that?

Remember the Simplicity of Stretching:

2—repetitions	2—sides, right and left
2—breaths' duration	2—hours between stretch time

Use relaxed stretches with no bouncing. Frequency is better than long periods of stretching.

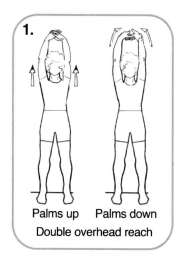

1.

Palms up   Palms down

Double overhead reach

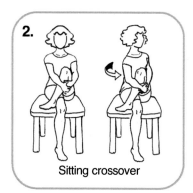

2.

Sitting crossover

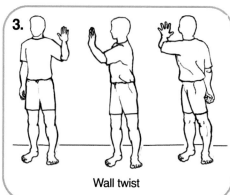

3.

Wall twist

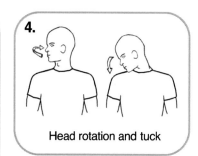

4.

Head rotation and tuck

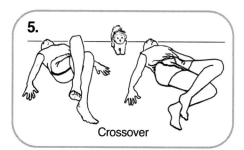

5.

Crossover

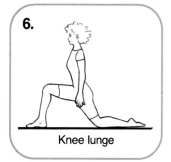

6.

Knee lunge

Please refer to **Appendix 1: Stretch Instructions** in the back of this book for more details on these stretches.

"BACKWARD LEAN" POSTURE

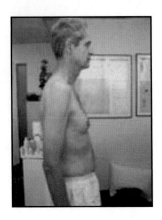 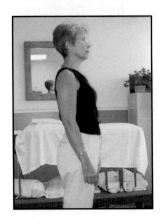 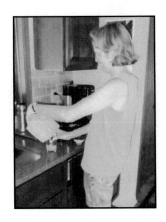

Whoa! Leaning backward is hard to do, yet it is common to see. How does it happen?

As muscles get tight in the low back and you try to keep your shoulders back, you begin to shift your weight to the heels and the body shifts backward.

What are the consequences of having a backward-leaning posture?

- To keep from falling backward, you tense the muscles in the front of your legs to help counter the backward lean.
- The head tends to come forward to counter the body's leaning backward and to help keep you balanced.
- The posture becomes habitual and begins to feel normal, straining muscles that respond in pain.

Several muscles tighten to cause pain when you are leaning backward:

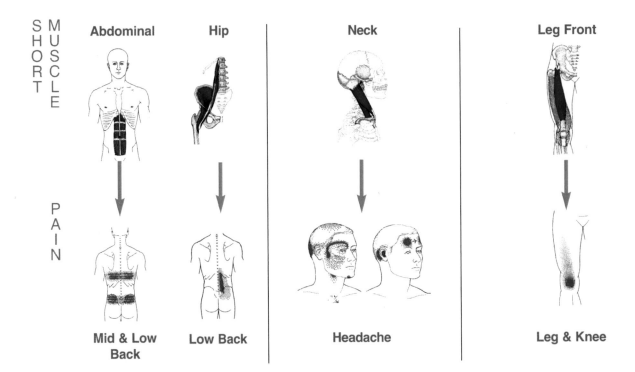

SHORT MUSCLE	Abdominal	Hip	Neck	Leg Front
PAIN	Mid & Low Back	Low Back	Headache	Leg & Knee

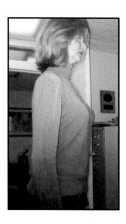

- Practice shifting your weight to the center or slightly to the front of your feet.
- You will probably feel like you will fall forward, but you won't.
- As you shift your weight forward, your head will automatically move back over your shoulders instead of jutting forward.
- Lift your head and chest as though you were a puppet with a string lifting you upward or taller.

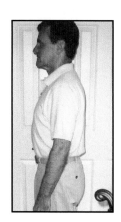

Corrected "Backward Lean" Posture

Stretches for reversing the muscle tightness resulting from the *backward lean* posture

THE RULE OF TWO APPLIES:
2 — Repetitions
2 — Breaths
2 — Hours
2 — Sides (both)

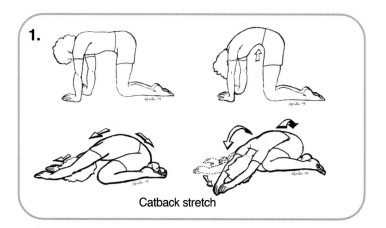

1.

Catback stretch

Practice posture changes in front of a mirror

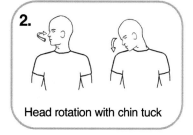

2.

Head rotation with chin tuck

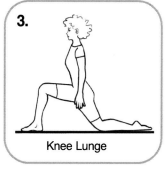

3.

Knee Lunge

F O C U S

- **Stretch gently, no hard pull.**
- **Hold the stretch steady with no bouncing.**

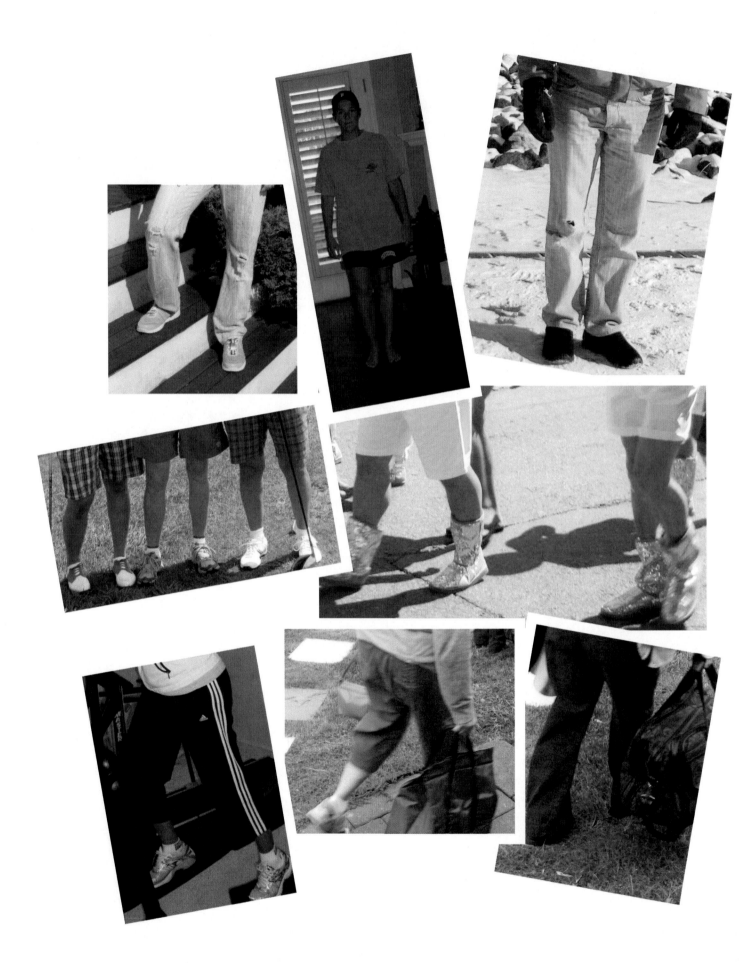

Chapter 5.
Walking: It Should Be Easy

I have had a lot of people contact me regarding their chronic pain. Sitting, standing, sleeping, and even walking had become painful. Walking should be easy, so automatic, that you just do it. But for many, walking has become difficult and painful.

Frustrated that walking has become an issue, people change shoes, and some even change socks. A few walk faster, and others slow down, walking only when they have to. The following patient scenarios illustrate some of the walking issues that can result in pain.

Carol. Carol called to see if I could help her get back to the daily walking she used to enjoy with a group of friends. "It seems I can walk around the house, but to go outside for a walk, oh no! I can't even walk a few blocks before tightness and discomfort makes me quit. I used to walk a couple of miles a day. What is going on?" she asked.

Obviously, something had changed: shoes, surface, walking mechanics, time, overload, something. "Tell me about your routine for the group walking," I said.

"Well, I get up at the last minute because we get together at 6:00 a.m. so we can walk before work. I grab my clothes and shoes, gulp down a cup of strong coffee, and off I go. I really feel pretty good when I start."

We checked her shoes, and they seemed to be good walking shoes. "Any stretching before you start?" I asked. I explained that starting the walk, basically straight from getting up, meant her muscles were still *waking up* also. They needed a chance to move a bit and warm up before being asked to start working. Muscles are always a little tighter in the morning because there has not been much movement during the night. Tight muscles often begin to ache if they aren't stretched and warmed up prior to using them.

"How about if I give you a few stretches to do before your walks? Offer them to your group as well. Perhaps all of you could spend some preparation time stretching before striding out for your walk. Spend a few minutes stretching after your walk also. The tightness you get in your muscles from the walk should not be carried to work and throughout the day."

Since Carol already experienced tight muscles and pain when walking, I suggested she do her stretches every couple of hours during the day for a few days before resuming the group walking. This would help to release some of her muscle tightness and allow the muscles to lengthen a bit more. Lengthening would help the muscles to move more easily on her extended walks.

"Muscles *learn* to stay where you repeatedly *put them,* "I explained. "They like stretching, and they'll function without tightness and strain if you routinely make stretching a part of the day." I also suggested Carol eat something before her walk, preferably with some protein as well as carbohydrates, to give her muscles some fuel.

Carol called several days later. "You won't believe it. I have a small shake with protein and fruit, I stretch out before meeting the others, then we all stretch a few minutes and off we go. Wow! What a difference it has made. All of us feel better, and we may even start walking further on the weekends. It is really fun walking again."

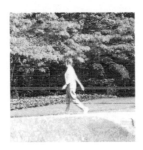

**Taking care of the little things
Opens your pathways
To more adventure!**

Tim. When Tim called to make an appointment to see me at the clinic, he must have been hurting a lot, since he said he was walking with a slight limp. He mentioned his feet hurt so badly he thought he might be getting *plantar fasciitis,* a painful inflammatory condition of the foot.

"I just don't get it," he said. "Walking is simply putting one foot in front of the other without even thinking. But, man, it's amazing how much it can hurt. I know I'm walking funny, just trying to lessen the pain, but I'm at a loss, since nothing is really working."

I asked Tim to bring several pairs of shoes that he wears frequently during an average week. I also wanted him to bring some photographs of sleep postures—not during sleep, just in the various postures he might use during the night—along with some sitting postures. We would look for the more common things that can cause foot and leg pain.

When Tim walked in, the first thing I noticed were the flip-flops he was wearing. We definitely had to talk about those. I hoped he didn't have too many sandals or shoes with open backs, but he did.

"Do you wear those flip-flops often, Tim?" I asked.

"No, not really, but I do have a couple of pairs of sandals, and some others that are similar. I wear them quite a bit at this time of year," he said.

"Let me give you an idea of what happens with *open-back shoes*."

- You have to grip with your toes to keep the sandals and flip-flops on your feet as you walk. That gripping *shortens* the muscles on the bottom of your foot every time you take a step. That can be the beginning of *plantar fasciitis,* a painful foot inflammation he mentioned when he initially called, as well as *foot and toe cramping.*

  The gripping with the toes can even be the beginning of *hammertoes,* where the toes stay curled under from the frequent gripping motion.

  Your heel tends to slide off to the side at the back of the shoe, since nothing is holding it in place. This position of your foot on the shoe can result in undue stress on the *Achilles tendon* and on *the stressed angle on your foot*, which changes muscle function. Severe strain can result in an Achilles tendon rupture."

- You cannot do a full foot roll of "heel to toe" when walking because it is difficult to keep on your shoe on if you do. Instead, you only *slightly lift the heel* of the back foot as you take a step, which lets you only *partially bend the knee*. This makes it necessary to *lift the hip* to have room to swing your leg forward. Such an altered step results in *hip and knee pain, stiff toes, and a painful arch."*

The issue is the *open back*. Any shoe you wear should have something to help hold the shoe on your foot, either a strap or a closed heel, to allow for a normal heel-to-toe walking motion.

Tim responded, "The slip-on shoes seem so easy to use, but I guess they really don't give me any support. I kind of knew that they weren't the best for me, but I was just being a bit lazy."

I suggested he try looking for a shoe that has some cushion as well, although you don't need the excessive cushioning often found in the heel of a running shoe. To find a flexible shoe, place one hand at the heel of the shoe and another at the toe. Push up on the toe to see if the shoe bends easily in the area where the ball of your foot would be. Twist it to be sure there is a slight resistance, not a "wet-noodle" feel. Walk around the store for ten or fifteen minutes as you look at other things, just to be certain the shoe is comfortable: no seams hitting in the wrong place, plenty of toe space, and no heel slipping.

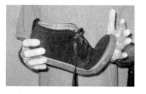
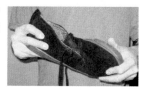

After addressing the shoes, we identified another issue for Tim from the pictures he brought to the appointment: he is a *stomach sleeper* who keeps his toes pointed as he sleeps. The muscles of his calves stay shortened when his toes are pointed for a number of hours every night. These tight muscles elicit pain that refers to the heel and the foot itself.

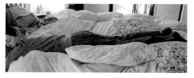

"Don't tell me I need to sleep on my back. I just can't get to sleep that way, no matter how hard I try. Could side sleeping work to give my legs and feet a posture that would let them relax a bit?" he asked.

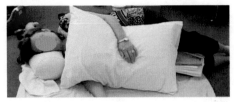

"Good choice," I said. "Just don't curl up when you get on your side. Keep your legs out fairly straight, with a pillow between your knees. That allows the hips, legs, and feet to be in a more neutral and relaxed posture. You'll find that your feet will be comfortable when you get up and take those first few steps in the morning. If you make these changes and do a couple of stretches throughout the day, you should be able to just walk again, without pain or even thinking about it."

With any walking you do, be aware when your feet hurt, tire easily, or are just uncomfortable.

Take time to figure out *why* this is happening, and why walking is not enjoyable. Look at your shoes, the way you are walking, how tight your leg muscles feel, and anything else that you could easily change to feel good.

The following section covers a number of issues that may make walking uncomfortable, issues that often result in foot and ankle pain, leg aching and cramping, and structural changes that can be devastatingly painful. Take a look and note the simple changes you can make once you know what to do.

Then come on, let's go take a walk!

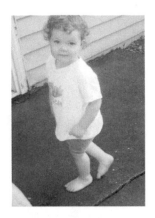 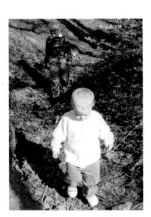 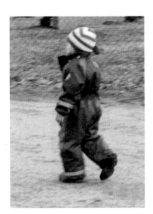

Feet—Our Foundation

Before we tackle shoes, let's look at feet. Your feet are forever under stress. What people do with their feet is unbelievable! Feet are the foundation of muscle movement. You use your feet constantly, and you are creating stress far beyond what you would imagine. Twenty-six small bones, with a lot of tendons attaching muscles to those bones, make up the structure of your feet. A majority of people will have some kind of foot problem during their lifetime. So what things do you need to know and do to avoid foot problems?

- *Feet are different when sitting, standing, and weight bearing; or in motion.*

- *Feet vary in size with temperature, humidity, and the time of day.*

- *Feet change, usually becoming larger as you age and as your foot muscles become bigger from use.*

Feet are complex, and the way you walk and the shoes you wear can either help or hurt your feet. They can aid in keeping your feet healthy or be significant factors in causing deformities of the bones and joints, as well as straining the muscles of your feet.

Feet usually experience more stress and wear than any other part of your body. True, they are made to handle their role of support and movement, and they do it well until you interfere. It is so common to compromise the natural state of your feet, altering their function by the shoes you wear, the way you walk, the weight you gain, the overload of work, lack of stretching and relaxation, and even lack of movement from sitting too much. Feet are certainly not designed to function without the help of shoes that not only fit your feet properly, supporting your bones and muscles, but also allow and encourage a good walking movement.

Feet are individual, unique to each person. Although we all basically have the same bones, muscles, and other tissues that comprise our feet, the way those parts are put together creates some interesting variations. Bone size and alignment, the shape and size of the muscles of the leg and foot, and muscle development are some of the factors that account for the differences. How you use, fail to use, or abuse your legs and feet throughout your life determines other differences between individuals. It is important to take the best care of your feet that you can: exercise and stretch your feet and toes.

Healthy feet must be helped out by the shoes you wear. Note that your feet do not perfectly match anyone else's feet. And yet shoes are manufactured hundreds or thousands at a time from the same mold. You need to be very careful to buy shoes *that fit you.*

Why do people buy shoes that don't fit? Here are some of the reasons I hear the most:

- They are cute.
- The color matches some of their outfits.
- They are in style this year.

- They make their feet look smaller.

- They are less expensive than some other styles.

- They are in a hurry and can't find the perfect pair anywhere, so these will do.

- They are easy to get in and out of.

- They have a hard time finding a shoe that fits, so they usually settle for whatever will work best.

It is no wonder some eighty percent of the population will at some point experience foot problems!

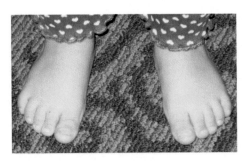

Happy, feel-good feet, go for it!

"Dudley Morton's Foot" or Long Second-Toe Joint

An Issue of Balance and Pain

Have you ever had a problem with balance when standing or moving around? What about achy legs and sore joints? You may have even noticed that it is difficult to get your body to relax as you are moving around. All of these situations can become chronic from a foot condition called *Dudley Morton's foot.* Simply put, for those with Morton's foot, the big toe joint (where the toe meets the foot) is further back than the position of the joint of the second toe. Although the tip of the second toe can be longer, appear slightly longer, or be at an even level with the tip of the big toe, it is *the joints where the toes are attached to the foot that are the issue.* The Morton's foot configuration makes you stand on a straight-line base of support when you are on your feet instead of having the foot supported on a tripod base, as is the case for the usual makeup of the foot, where the position of the toe joints slant down from the big toe. It is the difference between balancing on a bicycle (straight-line balance) and a tricycle (tripod balance).

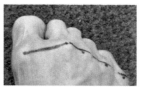

Toes are bent so you can see the toe joint

Dr. Dudley J. Morton wrote about this foot issue in the 1920s. Janet G. Travell, M.D. furthered the understanding of this condition, and came to recognize and teach that the long-second-toe-joint configuration could be the cause of chronic muscle pain throughout the body. Why is this?

The problem with a Morton's foot is that the body weight is not distributed across the bottom of the foot in a way that results in balanced posture and movement. Remember, Morton's foot affords only straight-line support for standing: from your heel to the joint of the second toe. Without a stable base in the feet, the muscles of the feet, legs, hips, and back must be constantly moving, rocking just slightly back and forth, and tightening or bracing in an attempt to keep you steady or balanced. This constant shifting puts undue stress on the joints, and also puts significant stress on the muscles. They can fatigue from this constant demand. As muscles fatigue, they tighten, and when they get too tight (or short), they begin to elicit pain. If not corrected, the strain from Morton's foot can result in ongoing chronic muscle pain.

Because foot structure is such an important issue in creating and maintaining balance, it is the key to the proficient movement of the body. Even though you may not recognize that you have a "balance" problem, you may still experience other common signs of the Morton's foot issue:

- *Fatigue or lack of energy.* Because more energy is required to maintain a sense of balance as you move about, you may tire easily.

- *Pain* as a result of the muscles shifting. You may notice symptoms in the feet, ankles, knees, hips, back, and upward through the shoulders.

- *Numbness and tingling in the feet* may or may not be a symptom.

- *Tendency toward weak ankles or easily "turning" or spraining your ankle joint.* Remember, you may be standing on a less stable base of support.

- *Calluses.* It is not unusual to find calluses (areas of thick and hardened skin), on the bottom of the foot under the second toe joint. This happens from the extra weight borne on the sole under that joint as you walk with your straight-line base of support: heel to a push-off at the second toe joint.

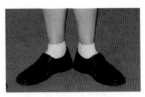

You may also find calluses on the outside of the big toe and the little toe as a result of the rocking/gripping of the foot as it tries to stay balanced. This constant rocking movement also causes friction against the shoe, which can result in calluses on the outer edges of the foot as well.

- *Feet turned out when standing or walking.* This is an attempt to create a wider base of support, more of a tripod stance or base. While this may slightly increase balance, it also rotates the hip outward and over time, shortens the hip rotator muscles. Do it enough, and the muscles begin to function from that rotated position more often: it can become their habit to function incorrectly. This can eventually result in hip and leg pain, as well as act as a stress on the hip joint itself.

Now you are thinking, "That is all fine and good, but if this foot thing is really a factor in my chronic pain, how can I tell if I have Morton's foot? Give me some direction for figuring it out."

Steps for Evaluating Dudley Morton's Foot/Long Second-Toe Joint

The difference may be subtle and difficult to observe, but these steps will help you with the evaluation. It is *not the length of the second toe that determines the condition; it is the joint where the toe meets the foot that needs to be evaluated.* To determine your foot structure, stand barefoot and do the following:

- *Look at the tips of the toes.* Is the second toe longer than the big toe? That makes it easy to determine if you have a Morton's foot. *If your second toe is longer than your big toe*, the joint *will* always be further ahead, and you do have a Morton's foot.

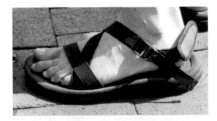

- Toe length may not always be the best way to determine if you have a Morton's foot, since it is the position of the *joints of the first and second toe that is important.* The difference may be subtle.

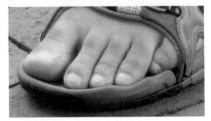

**Does he or doesn't he?
It is hard to tell.**

- To be sure, *bend the toes down and look, then feel with your finger, for the small bumps that indicate the end of the first and second toe bones.* Mark the centers of the bumps with a pen, and draw a line from the middle of the big toe bump the middle of the second toe bump. If the bone of the second toe is even slightly ahead of the first, you have a Morton's foot.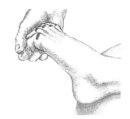

- *Separate the second and third toes. Look for extra skin or "webbing" between the two*, as compared to the space between the first and second toe and between the other toes. This is a common characteristic of a Morton's foot and another good indication of its presence.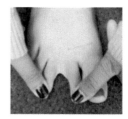

- Check for calluses on the areas of the feet mentioned earlier, such as on the bottom of the foot under the second toe joint.

If you do have a Morton's foot, what can you do about it? How can you correct it to improve balance and allow muscles throughout the body to relax as you move about?

Correction of the imbalance resulting from this foot structure involves adding some height or support under the ball of the big toe on the bottom of the foot. If you raise the joint of the big toe (commonly called the ball of the big toe), it shifts the weight off the long second-toe joint and allows all the toe joints to contact the ground, forming a tripod foundation. This improves your balance as you both stand and move about.

How is the correction accomplished? There are many products on the market, but most seem to be more complicated than what you need for the correction of Morton's foot. While other products may be useful, there are two that I have found to be easy to use and particularly helpful. They are pictured here:

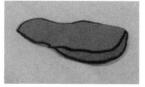

Solemate™

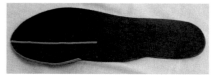

Posture Control Insoles®

The *Solemate™* is small and goes on your foot or inside the shoe (see photo below). The outer edge, under the ball of the foot, is raised. That moves the place where the foot contacts the ground forward, away from the second toe joint. This puts your point of walking contact on the first toe joint, and shifts and balances that joint with the fifth toe joint. All the toe joints are now in a weight-bearing position, which puts you in a stable tripod balance.

- *These little corrective inserts can attach to your foot* if you prefer wearing certain kinds of sandals, or if you insist on going barefoot. Barefoot, however, is not a good choice if you need a heel lift for leg length difference, as discussed in the previous chapter on standing.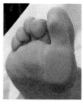

- The *Solemate*™ can also be attached to the underside of a shoe insert or insole. This makes it easier to use with sandals (closed-back sandals, of course.)

- If the shoe does not have a removable insole, you can attach the *Solemate*™ to the top of the insole.

ProKinetics® are another option useful for those with Morton's foot. These insoles have a built-in raised area from behind the big toe joint through to the end of the toe, so you are allowed to move through your step with full correction for Morton's foot. Many orthotics stop at the front end of the arch, offering arch support but 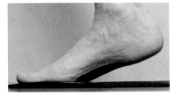 no correction for Morton's foot under the ball of thebig toe. Besides correcting Morton's foot, the *ProKinetics*® insert will also, to some extent, address the issue of the foot's rolling inward: two corrections in one comfortable insole.

Note: Sources for ordering *Solemates*™ and *ProKinetics*® (with or without arch supports) may be found in the *Contact and Product Resources* appendix.

There are also a couple of easy corrections that you can do yourself that have significant results.

Corrective Option 1:

- Buy a pair of full-length foam inserts. Any insert will work, but ones that are a little heavier or thicker will last longer and be a little more comfortable. The insole should be wide enough so that it does not slide sideways within the shoe. This may require many people to use men's insoles to ensure proper fit.

- Cut out the insole under the second, third, fourth, and fifth toe joints, leaving the rest of the insole under the entire foot, including the big toe, as shown in the photo. Notice that because the insole remains under the first/big toe, it is raised higher than the second and remaining toes. The rest of the insert stops short of the heads of the other toe joints. Remember, the insole should be wide enough that it does not slide around inside the shoe.

The insole you have created with the cut-out sets the first/big toe somewhat further from the ground than the second toe and the other toe joints. The pressure, as you place your foot to walk, is on the elevated first joint, and shifts to the fifth toe joint, putting you on a tripod base of support. The second toe joint is lowered out of the way.

This option mimics the structure of the *ProKinetics®* described earlier.

Corrective Option 2:

- Buy some adhesive felt; that is, felt with a sticky back. Sources may be found in the *Resources and Contacts* appendix.

- Cut a strip of adhesive felt wide enough to cover the joint of the big toe and long enough to cover the toe when it is in a slightly bent position, as shown in the photo. This option is similar to the Solemate™ described earlier.

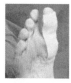

- If your shoe has an insole, remove it and place the felt into your shoe, carefully covering the entire area of the toe and joint of the big toe. You should be able to feel an indentation in the bottom of your shoe made by the pressure of the big toe.

  Note: if your shoe does not have a removable insole, this option is more difficult to place and position with certainty. You may have to try various placements of the felt in the area of the big toe to effect a favorable correction.

For those who discover they have Morton's foot, using these corrections will surprise you with the improved balance, whole-body relaxation, muscle relief, and movement ease they afford. Simple, but so very effective!

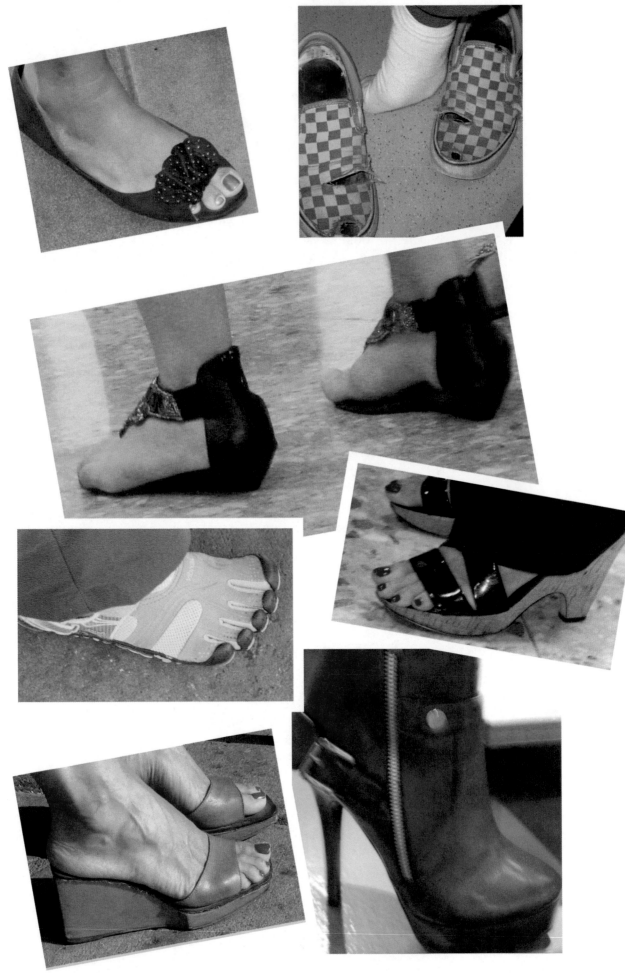

Chapter 6.
Shoes: What an Interesting Adventure

Shoes come in styles I could never have dreamed up. Few fit well, and you know some are probably not the best for you. But, well, you buy them anyway. Sometimes you aren't sure what is good because you have heard a lot of conflicting information about styles. There is so much information out there: from manufacturers, advertising, endorsements by important athletes, store "experts," and even doctors.

A lot of the information, when you think about it, probably goes against your own understanding and thinking. Remember, a great deal of the information presented to you is fashion driven, designed for visual appeal. You are told that as long as shoes are *comfortable* at the store, it is okay, even when those same shoes have added pads, heel cushions, and are stretched before you even pay for them. But, oh, they do look so good on your foot.

As an example, I took my fifteen-year-old niece to the shoe store for some Keds®- type shoes that had sparkling stuff all over them. She thought they were "soooo cool," and everyone was wearing them! When I picked up the shoe to check it out, I found that the sole was so stiff it did not bend at all. I mentioned this to the store clerk, and his comment was: "Oh, I know, they don't bend at all; they are just a fashion shoe, but kids love them." Kids were buying them like crazy, but they couldn't even take one normal step in them. Whew!

Ill-fitting shoes affect your entire body.

If your feet hurt:

- *You change how you walk,* from a normal gait to more extreme motions: flat-footed steps, short or tiny steps, slapping your foot down as you step, turning your feet outward, rolling them inward, bending your body forward, keeping the knees bent, tilting your pelvis, jutting your head forward, and rounding your shoulders.

- *You change how far you walk,* decreasing the distance because of fatigue or discomfort, although you need the exercise.

- *You change how you stand.* You shift and change your position, lean against something for support, bend one knee, or kick one leg out to the side, resulting in muscle fatigue and unnecessary strain.

- *You engage other muscles* not normally involved in standing or walking to help you move or stay balanced. You swing the leg or foot to the side, hike your hip, or move your leg forward.

- The list goes on . . . every compromise or adaption of movement you make because of your shoes could eventually lead to pain and foot deformity. Think twice, or even three times, before you buy that next pair of shoes!

Remember, there is no one best shoe or style of shoe. There are so many varieties available, and retailers hope that you will select one, even if it isn't really what you wanted and doesn't necessarily fit. The best shoe *fits you* without causing undue stress on your feet: it has good support, cushioning, bends easily, has lots of toe room, is comfortable, and works for what you want to wear it for. It can be a daunting search, but don't give up.

Look over the shoe section of this book and decide to be really good to your feet by getting shoes that fit in every way. I've given you a whole list of successful buying tips. You may even have more to add.

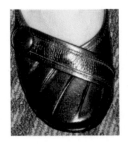 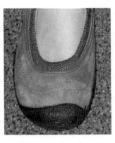 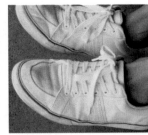 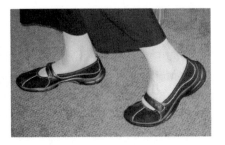

Here are some well-fitting shoes with all the right pieces.

SHOE STYLES

There are many different shoe styles. I will focus on some you see a lot of people wearing, and that can cause problems. On the left, I describe how the style of shoe can affect your body and how it can determine walking movement. On the right, you will see the pain pattern that can result.

Stiff and Inflexible Shoes

Cumulative Pain Results

■ **Limited ankle movement,** so you tend to roll off the tip of the shoe instead of bending the toes. **Increased calf contraction/shortening.**

Leg, foot, and heel pain

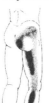

■ **Limited knee and hip motion** when ankle motion is restricted.

Hip and leg pain, and mimics "Sciatica"

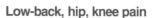

■ **Little or no toe bend on push-off** of the back foot when walking. **Hiking the hip** or **swinging the leg to the side** are common compensations as you bring the leg forward.

Low-back, hip, knee pain

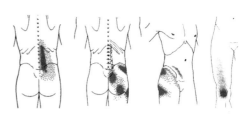

■ **Restricted ankle and knee motion,** limiting calf and Achilles tendon movement. Strain and calf cramping can result in pain.

Leg and foot pain

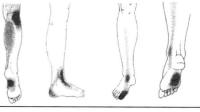

■ **Limited movement** of the muscles on the **bottom of the feet.**

Stiff, painful toes and toe joints

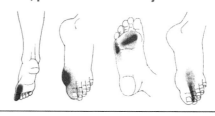

■ Tendency for **flat gait** – little heel-toe motion.

All of the above types of pain may be experienced.

Shoes stiff = muscles short = joints stiff = PAIN

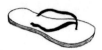

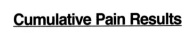

Open-Back Shoes

- **Gripping with toes** to keep shoes on.

Cumulative Pain Results

Stiff, painful feet and toes

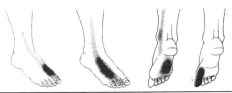

- **Gripping** shortens the muscles on the top and bottom of the foot and the shins.

Foot pain

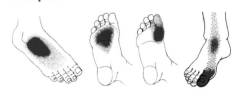

- **Partial heel lift** on rolling motion of heel-toe walking movement.

Leg, knee, calf, and heel pain

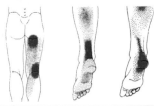

- **Limited heel raise** results in **hip hiking** to make room to swing leg forward in the walking motion.

Hip, buttock and leg pain

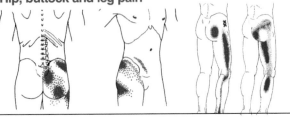

- **Foot is often free to slide to side** and often settles off to the side of shoe.

Calf and foot pain and cramping

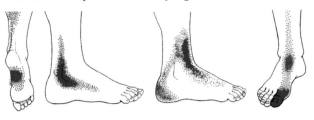

- Open-back shoe often has big toe box allowing **foot to slide** around with additional **toe gripping.**

Heel and foot pain

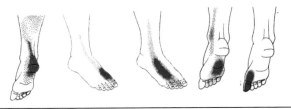

- Open-back shoe **can have a narrow toe box** to help keep the shoe on but **squishes the toes** together.

Any and all of the above pain may be experienced, as well as nerve pain.

Pointed-Toed Shoes

Cumulative Pain Results

- Narrow toe box **squishes the toes** into a small area.

Stiff, painful feet and toes

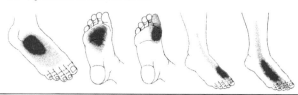

- Pointed shoe tapers quickly, causing **undo force or pressure** on the foot.

Foot pain, swelling, and enlargement of joints (bunions)

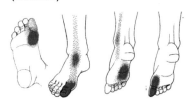

- **Bunching** of the foot from too little room.

Foot pain and nerve irritation and inflamation (neuromas)

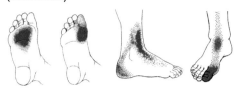

- Small pointed toe causes **gripping** with toes for balance, since the full foot is not in contact with the shoe bottom. This can result in decreasing balance when you stand and walk.

Painful feet and toes

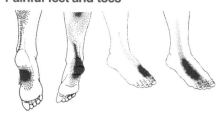

- **Foot and toe compensation** from small and tapered toe box.

Pain on tips and sides of toes (ingrown nails & calluses)

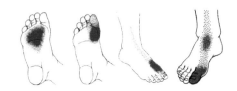

High-Heeled Shoes

- **Shorten calf muscles** to extent it may be painful to wear flatter shoes.

Cumulative Pain Results

Calf, Achilles tendon, and heel pain

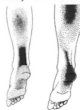

- The **knees stay flexed** and the **shin tends to turn inward,** resulting in a torque and undue pressure on the inside of the knee.

Knee, ankle, and toe pain

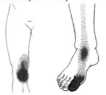

- **Unnaturally shifts weight forward,** resulting in undue pressure on the front of the foot, forcing **bones to become irregularly shaped.**

Leg, foot, and toe pain

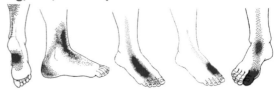

- Forward weight shift tilts the pelvis and mis-positions the low back, thereby losing the lumbar shock-absorbing function.

Low-back, hip, and leg pain

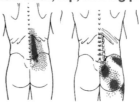

- Shifting the weight forward causes you to **lean forward, flattens the low back,** and **moves the head and mid back backward,** in an effort to balance the body.

Neck, shoulder, and back pain

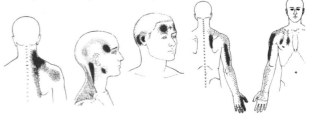

- Often have narrow or pointed toe box, **squishing the toes.**

Foot and toe pain, as well as frequent nerve pain

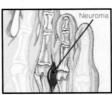

indypodiatry.com

Inflammed and swollen nerve

High-Heeled Shoes, continued

■ Shifting your weight forward and balancing on a small point of contact on the heel **decreases balance,** resulting in turning your feet out for stability.

Cumulative Pain Results

Lower leg, ankle, and foot pain

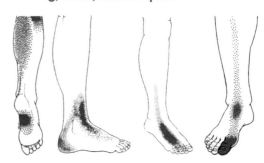

■ **Limited length of stride** reduces leg movement at the hip.

Hip and low-back pain

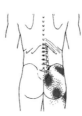

■ **Limited heel-toe motion** results in a **flat gait and hip hiking** to make room to swing the leg forward in the walking motion.

Hip, buttock, and leg pain

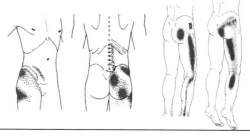

■ **Constricts calf muscle,** decreasing its action as an "auxiliary pump" returning blood to the heart.

Calf pain and cramping

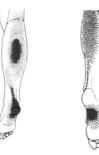

WHAT CAN SHOES DO TO YOU?

Shoes are often *fashion-driven,* and what you buy often goes against even your own common sense. Why would you buy, let alone wear, shoes that can do the following to your feet?

Bunions

Narrow or pointed-toed shoes leave you in a situation you are not going to win. These, shoes *squish* the toes in, up and over and under each other and put a lot of *pressure* on the big and little toe joints. **High-heeled shoes** increase the *pressure* on the bottom of the foot as well. Both shoe styles can cause deformities such as bunions. The added *pressure* on the front of the foot from being bunched up often results in the toes *gripping* for balance and stability. This gripping, in turn, increases the possibility of bunions. Select shoes with a low heel and a wide, more rounded toe box.

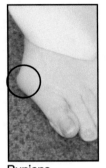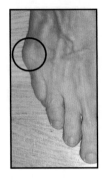

Bunions

Calluses, Corns, and Blisters

As bunions develop, the positions of the toes change, which can increase *pressure* on other bony parts of foot, resulting in calluses and corns.

Narrow or pointed-toed shoes and low toe box shoes *don't leave enough room* for all of the toes to have flat contact with the sole of the shoe. It is common to find a pointed-toed shoe style with **high heels**. The toes are *squished* together, *rubbing* on each other or rubbing on the sides and tops of the shoes, creating *friction* that can result in calluses, blisters, and corns. If the shoes are tight at the heel, the *rubbing* can create calluses and blisters.

Shoes that are **too short** can cause the end of the toes to *rub* at the tip of the shoe and create calluses and bruises.

Likewise, shoes that are *too wide and without good support* such as **open-back shoes, sandals, and slip-ons** can leave you *gripping* with your toes to keep your foot steady or balanced. This can create calluses on the toes and on the outer edges of your foot. Being loose at the heel, allowing foot movement up and down, can result in additional blisters.

Leather that is too stiff or hard, **wrinkled socks or thick seams in your socks or shoes** can cause *friction* that also results in blisters. Put your foot and shoe side by side. The shoe should be slightly bigger than your foot in every way.

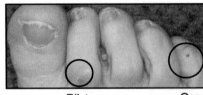

Blister   Corn

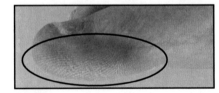

Callus

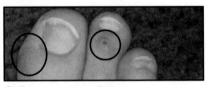

Callus   Corn

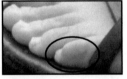

Callus

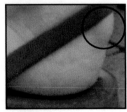

Callus

Hammertoes and Mallet Toes

Open-back shoes are difficult to walk in without *gripping* with the toes with every step to keep the shoe on the foot. Toe *gripping* is also seen with **high-heeled shoes,** as you strive for better balance. That constant gripping shortens the muscles and their tendons on the bottom of the foot, resulting in the toes being drawn up. It becomes harder to straighten the toes, and eventually, they stay bent. It is called a hammertoe if the bend is at the middle toe joint, and a mallet toe if the bend is at the joint nearest the tip of the toe.

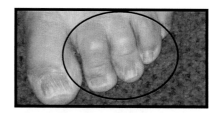
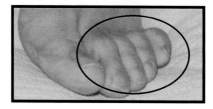

Hammertoes

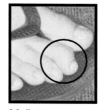
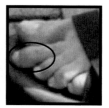

Mallet toe

This *curling* in, or *gripping*, of the toes can occur when the shoe is **too short**, not leaving enough room at the end of the shoe for the toes to lie flat, resulting in hammertoes. The toes can also *hang off* the front of an open-toed shoe, resulting in gripping for balance when walking.

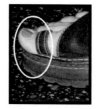
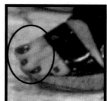

Toes off edge can result in gripping

Achilles Tendon Strain

Open-back shoes in many cases offer little support. The heel of the foot is allowed to *move back and forth* on the shoe, the heel frequently settling in an off-center position on the shoe. This can lead to the *bowing* of the Achilles tendon because of the angle of the heel. This is a common occurrence with most **open-back shoes** and can result in a very painful experience, often making the tendon vulnerable to a rupture injury. Shoes must have either a strap or an enclosed heel to allow your foot to function with support and balance and to be capable of a normal heel-toe walking motion.

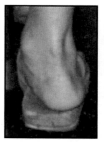
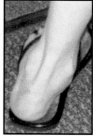

Bowed achilles in teenagers

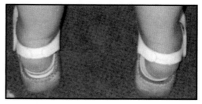

Bowed achilles in adult

143

Plantar Fasciitis

Stiff, rigid, inflexible shoes *don't allow normal movement of the foot* when walking, which often results in *plantar fasciitis*, an inflammatory condition on the bottom of the foot that is extremely painful. The fascia, which is right under the skin and covers the muscles, gathers and attaches near the heel. When this tissue is continually shortened from toe *gripping* with **open-back shoes** or stressed by a *hard pull* from wearing **high-heeled shoes**, a small tear can occur at the attachment. The tighter the foot tissue becomes, the more the pain is experienced. Often the worst pain is the first step out of bed in the morning, since the tissue has shortened from non-use during the night. The healing process can be lengthy, since you are on your feet during the day, continuing to irritate and stress the foot. Correctly fitting shoes are a must: flexible, low heeled, supportive, with a wide rounded or squared toe box. No stiff, non-bending shoes!

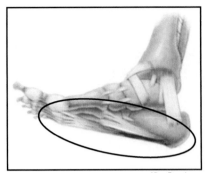

King Brand.com

Inflammation

Toes Twisted or Crossed Under Other Toes

Narrow toe box shoes, while fashionable, do not allow for the toes to fully rest on the sole of the shoe. Once again **high-heeled shoes** can be the culprits for foot deformities and the pain involved. Left in a *crowded space*, the toes have little choice but to curl in, or to be pushed inwards, towards the center of the shoe. They often curl right under the toe next to them. It is not uncommon to see the 4th and 5th toes curled and often somewhat twisted from being forced into a narrow shoe. This curled position often affects balance, and abnormally pressured areas can develop calluses and corns. The lack of space between the toes leaves little air circulation and can result in fungal growth. You just cannot win with narrow shoes that have your feet bulging out the sides, or squished beyond recognition.

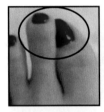
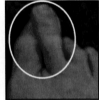
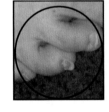
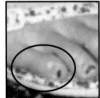

144

Neuromas

Narrow, pointed-toed shoes, and especially **high-heeled shoes**, continue their impact on the feet with nerve compression, resulting from toes *crammed* into a small space. The *unnatural weight bearing* may promote the development of a neuroma. Compression of the nerves that lie between the toes can result in inflammation and swelling. The most significant *compression* is usually on the middle toes, as the others are all pushed towards the narrow center of the shoe. A neuroma is a very painful condition often requiring surgery.

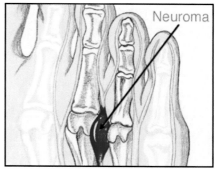

indypodiatry.com

Inflammed and swollen nerve

Ingrown or Cracked Toenails

Once again, **narrow, pointed-toed shoes** or **low toe box shoes** and the added forefoot pressure from **high-heeled shoes** can cause a problem of ingrown toenails. It is most common on the big toe, but can also be seen on the little toe, as a great deal of pressure is exerted on the toenail by these shoes. This results in the corner of the nail growing inward, becoming painful, swollen, and often inflamed.

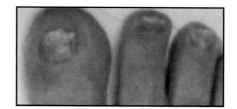

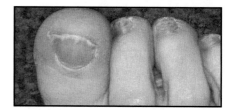

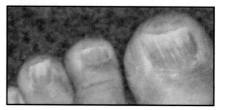

If you could eliminate any or all of the above foot deformities and pain complications just by wearing shoes that really fit your feet, why wouldn't you?

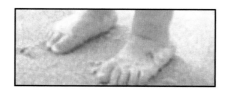

SHOE BUYING TIPS

Buy the shoe that *fits you*.
Don't go by what you had before.
Keep about ½" of room between the toes
and the end of the shoe.

Standing, draw your foot on a sheet of paper.
Set a shoe you want on top of the drawing. Does
the shoe cover all of the foot? If any of your
drawing shows, the shoe IS NOT FOR YOU!

Shoes must be flexible and bend easily.
Test the shoe by grabbing each end with your hands
and twisting in opposite directions. The shoe should
bend or twist where the ball of the foot would be.

Ball of foot should be at the widest part of the shoe,
where the curve of the sole begins.

All toes should rest on the shoe floor, should be
comfortable, and not bulging at the sides.

You should be able to wiggle all the toes up and
down within the shoe

Heel should have no slipping in the shoe, no
riding up and down. If the heel slips, don't just
go down half a size. You may need another
style of shoe.

Don't buy tight shoes and expect them
to "stretch out."

Ensure the shoe fits. No part of the foot
should be off the front edge of the shoe,
off the side of the shoe, nor push through
any cutout gaps.

Shoe top should be a soft, flexible
material that matches the shape of
the foot. Hard leather irritates bone
and skin.

Soles should be rough or have
tread, not smooth so as not
to be slippery

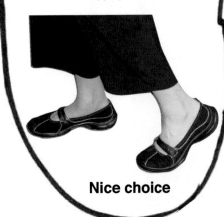

Nice choice

MORE SHOE BUYING TIPS

Try shoes on both the right and left foot.
Feet are often slightly different sizes, or
shoes may not be quite symmetrical.

Walk, jog, or run in the store to get a feel for the
shoe on your feet.

Wear socks, inserts, or orthotics you are most likely
to wear with this particular style of shoe. Select shoes
with removable insoles so you can easily modify or replace
them with orthotics if necessary.

Try a couple of different models and sizes
to make a good comparison. Don't rush
your decision.

**Lacing area and tongue should have some
padding**, especially if you have any bony
protrusions on the top of your foot. Laced
shoes should hold the foot firmly, but
comfortably. You know, they should feel "snuggly."

Fit shoes in the afternoon or after a workout,
when the feet may have swollen slightly. Feet
can swell as much as a full size during
aggressive activity.

The best shoe is one of real comfort,
not price or brand determined.

Don't buy a shoe you have to "break in"
before it is comfortable.

Heel counter should fit snugly so there
is neither excess movement nor space.
Note where the top of the heel
structure hits your foot. Resting too
high on the foot can cause blisters.

Check the quality of the shoe.
Set it on a flat surface near eye level.
The mid-line of the heel should be straight
up and down to the surface the
shoe is sitting on.
There should be no tilt to one side
or the other.
This allows the foot to be level in the shoe.

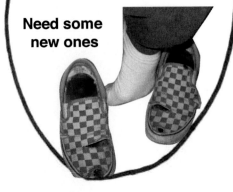

**Need some
new ones**

It is important
to understand that
the information
provided is of
a basic educational
nature only, and
does not constitute
medical advice
nor should it
replace medical
consultations
or advice.

Chapter 7.
Summary

Chronic pain—you used to ask "How did I get this way?" You have just seen a clear view of how many little daily uses of your muscles can be the answer to that question. Each mis-cue to your muscles has led them to develop incorrect ways of functioning. Together they became pieces of the puzzle that is your *chronic pain*.

You have been introduced to *simple changes* that can begin to reverse your chronic pain as soon as you begin practicing them.

Stretches that have been presented will further establish new patterns of muscle function and will continue to keep you pain free.

What a golden opportunity for you to take control and begin a revitalized lifestyle, one that expands all the activities, travel, relaxation, and fun-filled living that you have been wanting. You only need to choose to take the journey. I am here to help in any way I can. Enjoy your new life!

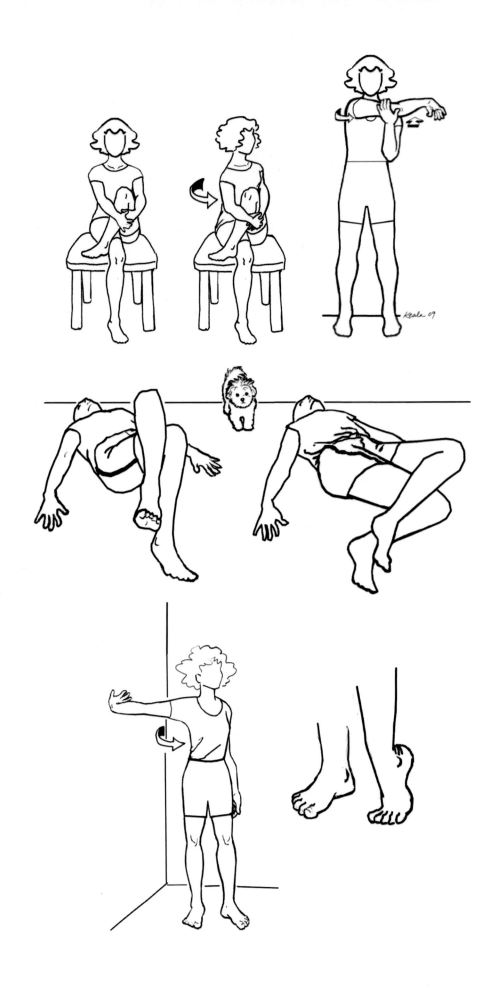

Appendix 1.
Stretch Instructions

Why you stretch has been addressed throughout this book.

How you stretch is also important, and stretch tips and focus points have been presented in each section of the book.

This appendix presents more detailed information on how to perform each stretch to make it as beneficial as possible. While there are many other beneficial stretches you can do, those chosen for this book are designed to aid in teaching muscles new patterns of function that will help eliminate your pain.

The stretches given are meant as part of the total program presented in this book and are to be used along with all other aspects of the book. They are to be performed as part of teaching muscles a new muscle memory, allowing muscles to function without the tightness that contributes to chronic pain. While an attempt has been made to allow the stretches to be used by everyone, if you have any special needs or concerns, it is important that you consult with your physician before beginning this program.

The stretches are grouped according to body parts they benefit. Muscles rarely function alone, but rather in groups, as they perform movements. Although the muscles have been grouped, there will obviously be overlaps among the muscles affected. It simply means that some stretches may be good for several areas of the body. This can enhance their effectiveness.

Focus Points:
- Stretches should be comfortable.
- Only stretch to the point of a slight pull. As muscles learn to be longer, you will be able to move further with your stretches without strain.
- It is better to *under-stretch* than to *over-stretch*.
- Hold the stretch steady, with no bouncing.
- Relaxed breathing gives the best results when stretching.

If you are tight and a stretch is difficult, start at a place where you feel no discomfort, just a gentle pull. As the muscle learns the new movement, you will be able to stretch further without forcing the muscles. This may take several days, which is fine. It is better to increase the stretch gradually to avoid stretching too hard and creating a muscle strain.

Rule of Two:
2 — Repetitions of each exercise.
2 — Breaths are taken before releasing the stretch.
2 — Sides of the body, one side at a time, to create a balance throughout the body.
2 — Hours before repeating the stretches.

All stretch movements should be performed at a normal, smooth pace. There is a *natural momentum to movement*. Stretching slowly (in anticipation of pain) requires you to tense muscles against that natural momentum of muscle movement. Since you are trying to teach *new muscle memory,* you don't want to be tensing the muscles when you are teaching a *new muscle-elongated position* with stretching. The freer the movement, the more easily muscles will move, eliminating the pain factor.

Neck and Head

Face:

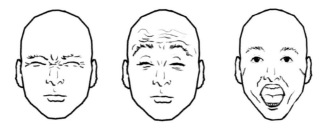

- Close your eyes as tight as you can.
- Relax your eyes but keep them closed, then raise your eyebrows as high as you can.
- Relax your eyes and open your jaw as wide as is comfortable.

Neck – Rotation:

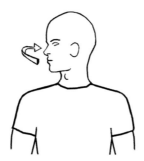

- Keeping your head level or chin slightly lowered, turn your head to the right as far as is comfortable.
- Keeping the same head position, turn your head to the left.

Neck – Rotation with tuck:

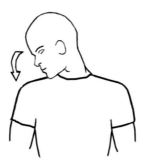

- Once again, turn your head comfortably to the right, and then gently tuck your chin toward the chest. (No cheating by opening the mouth to get the chin lower.)
- Repeat, turning your head to the left and lowering chin to chest.

Upper Body

Shoulders – Arm pull-down in front of body:

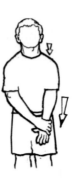

- Grasp one arm at the wrist.
- Keeping that arm straight, gently pull it down in front of you, *allowing your shoulder to lower* or drop as you do this. (The movement is similar to slowly reaching for the floor, but the arm can be relaxed since it is being guided by the pull-down).
- The head remains straight and relaxed.

Shoulders – Arm pull-down behind the body:

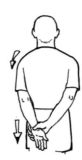

- Repeat the arm and shoulder pull-down, but this time with the arm behind the body.
- This should be a smooth, gentle pull, not a quick jerky motion.
- The head again remains straight.

Shoulders – Arm pull-down behind and across the body:

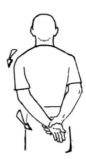

- Repeat the arm and shoulder pull-down with the arm behind the body.
- As the arm is pulled down, increase the angle to direct the arm and hand toward the opposite buttock.

Shoulders – Arm pull behind the back at waist level:

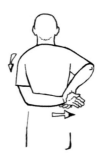

- Grasp one wrist behind the back with the opposite hand.
- Keeping the upper arm against your body, bend that arm at the elbow and bring it to waist level. (If the elbow moves away from the body or sticks out to the side, it will be difficult to bring the arm across the waist.)
- Pull the arm across the body at waist level to further lower the shoulder and lengthen the shoulder and neck muscles.
- The head remains straight ahead.

Shoulder – Arm pull across front of body:

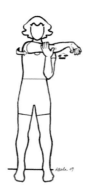

- With one hand, hold the opposite arm just above the elbow.
- Gently pull the arm across the front of the body.
- Keep the elbow straight as you bring the arm across and inward toward the chest.

Shoulder – Rotation:

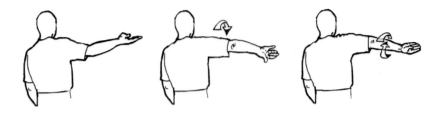

- Raise one arm out to the side to shoulder height. If it is painful to do this, lower the arm until it is at a comfortable height.
- Hold the arm in a palm-up position.
- Turn or roll the arm forward, moving the hand to another palm-up position.
- Reverse the movement, rolling the arm back to the original position.

Arms – Triceps, back of upper arm:

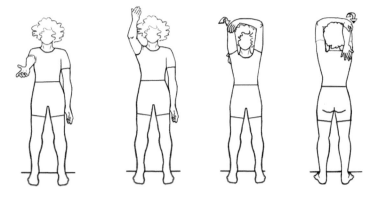

- Reach one arm out in front of you, palm of hand up.
- Bend at the elbow and place palm on shoulder, allowing the forearm to touch your face.
- With the opposite hand, grasp the elbow and slowly lift the bent arm overhead.
- Keep the arm next to the face, with the elbow following a straight line: *you should not be able to see your forearm as the bent arm is lifted overhead.*

Arms – Biceps, front of the upper arm:

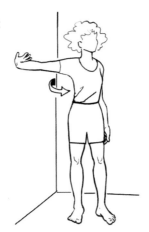

- Stand sideways next to a solid surface: a wall, closed door, tree, post, or something similar. Place your hand, palm flat, on the surface at shoulder height.
- The fingers should be pointing backward, thumb pointing up.
- If there is more than a slight pull anywhere along the arm, move the arm further back as though you were reaching behind you.
- As the stretch becomes easier, gradually slide the hand forward a little at a time, until the arm is straight out at shoulder height. This may take several days to accomplish.
- When, and only when, you feel no stretch with the arm at shoulder height, turn your upper body slightly away from the extended arm.

Arms – Biceps, front of the upper arm, version 2:

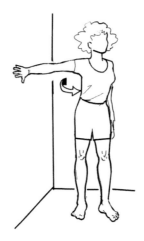

- Repeat the bicep stretch above, but with the palm on the flat surface in a thumb-down position.
- Remember to move the hand back if there is more than a slight stretch (pull).
- When your arm is straight at shoulder height, and you no longer feel a stretch in your arm or hand, turn your body slightly away from the extended arm.

Forearms and Hands – Reverse forearm:

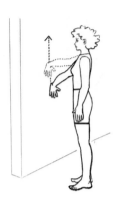

- Stand facing a solid surface: a wall, closed door, tree, post, or something similar. Place your hand, palm flat, on the surface, with the fingers pointing downward.
- Start with the hand placed below waist height.
- When you no longer feel a stretch at one level, move the hand upward about an inch. Over several days of repetitions performed every two hours, the stretch range will increase until the hand is straight in front of you at shoulder height.

Chest – Large arm circle backward:

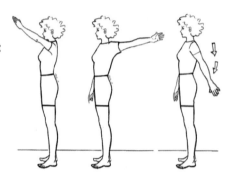

- With a straight but relaxed arm, reach arm forward and continue circling through a full backward circle, as though you were doing a swimming backstroke.
- If the arm and shoulder are tight, you will simply make a smaller circle, not reaching quite as high. That is fine. The circle will get bigger as the muscle stretch range increases.

Chest – Doorjamb:

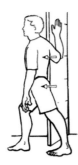

- Stand in a doorway with your hip even with the doorjamb (frame).
  Place the leg closest to the doorjamb in a step-forward position.
- The other leg is in a step-back position.
- Place your hand just above shoulder height, with your entire lower arm on the doorjamb: elbow, forearm, and hand.
- Bend your forward knee, slightly shifting your weight forward and beginning a stretch in the upper chest.
- As the stretch becomes easier, increase the knee bend, shifting your body forward and increasing the stretch.

Chest – Doorjamb, version 2:

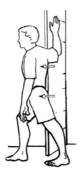

- Repeat the chest stretch above, changing only the placement of the forearm.
  The elbow is now placed *at* shoulder height, with the forearm resting on the doorjamb.
- Shift your weight forward as before to stretch the middle chest muscles.

Chest – Doorjamb, version 3

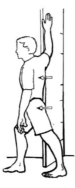

- Repeat the chest stretch above, changing again to a new placement of the forearm.
- The arm is now extended upward above head level, with the forearm still resting on the doorjamb.
- Shift your weight forward as before to stretch the lower chest muscles.

Back and Torso

Torso – Wall twist:

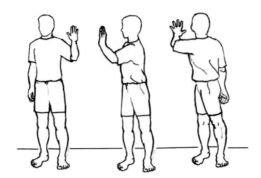

- Stand with your back to a wall, tree, fence, or something similar.
- Place your feet shoulder width apart.
- Twist the hips and reach with your outside arm to the wall behind you. Twist to the right and reach with the left arm. The other arm stays relaxed at your side.
- Repeat the twist to the left, reaching with the right arm.
- Stop the motion when you begin to feel a slight stretch anywhere.
- There should be no strain on the knees. You may bend them slightly if needed.
- The range of the twist increases as the muscles learn to stretch freely.
- When a full twist and reach is accomplished, you can reach higher with the arm to increase the stretch through the torso area.

Torso – Side bend:

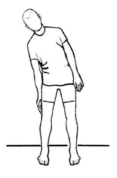

- Stand with your feet comfortably apart.
- Let your arms hang freely at your side.
- Lean sideways, allowing the hand to slide down the outside of your leg.
- Avoid leaning or bending forward—anatomically, you won't be able to lean very far to the side.
- You may feel the stretch anywhere along your side, as far down as into the hip.

Torso – Double overhead reach:

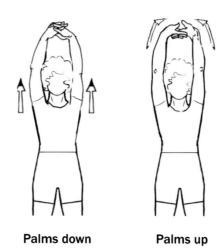

Palms down   Palms up

- Stand with feet shoulder width apart.
- Clasp hands in front of body with fingers laced.
- Reach both arms overhead with palms down.
- Decrease the reach if you feel more than a gentle stretch or pull anywhere.
- Bring arms to starting position.
- Repeat overhead reach with palms turned upward.
- Return to start position.

Torso – Overhead reach with side lean:

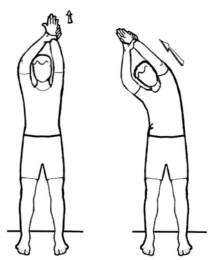

- Stand with feet shoulder width apart.
- Grasp one wrist with the opposite hand.
- Bring the arm overhead, increasing the reach with a gentle pull on the arm from the wrist.
- If you feel a stretch or pull from the arm reach, do not try to bring the arm higher. That will happen easily as the muscles learn to stretch.
- Once you can reach with the arm pull and you feel no stretch, lean your body slightly to the opposite side to increase the stretch on the muscles.

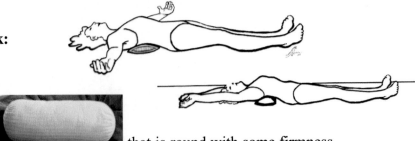

Torso – Pillow behind back:

- Select a roll pillow 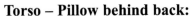 that is round with some firmness.
- Lying on your back, position the pillow across the shoulder blade area. The top of the pillow will be even with the armpit.
- The head should reach back to touch the floor. If this is painful, place a small folded towel behind the head.
- Place the arms out to the side at about shoulder height. As the stretch becomes easier, move the arms toward the head, and then overhead.
- The body across the pillow stretches the chest and abdominal muscles. Easy breathing eases the muscles into relaxation.

Torso – Butterfly:

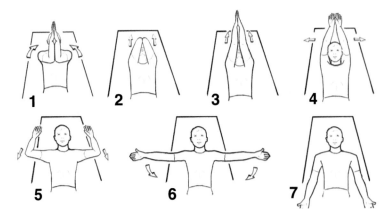

- This stretch is shown lying on the floor. It can also be performed in a standing position.
- Bring your arms together at shoulder height with elbows, forearms, and palms touching (1).
- Holding this position, reach the arms overhead, keeping the elbows together as long as you can (2).
- When the elbows begin to separate, straighten the arms and reach overhead as far as possible, palms still together (3).

When lying down, the arms are resting on the floor for the rest of the sequence.

- Keep arms extended overhead, and turn the arms and palms outward (4).
- With the elbows leading, bend the arms and bring them to shoulder height at a 90° angle (5). The arms and hands are still resting on the floor.
- Leading with the hands, circle with straight arms to bring the arms down (6).
- Complete the sequence with the arms at the side, palms up (7).

This stretch rotates the mid-back muscles on the shoulder blades and the chest muscles.

Back and Hip – Catback:

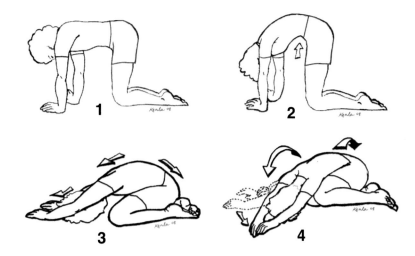

- Take a hands-and-knees position on the floor (1).
- Lower your head and round your back upward (2).
- Keeping the head tucked, shift back to sit on your heels. If this is uncomfortable for your knees, limit how far you do the sit-back (3a).
- Extend the arms forward (3b).
- Return to the start and the rounded-back position.
- This time, shift back at an angle to sit on the right heel (4a).
- Extend the arms forward and to the left, opposite the right-heel sitting position (4b). *Many of the back muscles are positioned at an angle; therefore they must be stretched at an angle. A straight shift back stretches only some of the muscles.*
- Return to the start and the rounded-back position.
- Shift back to sit on the left heel, with the arms extended and reaching to the right.

This stretch involves a number of muscles, so you may feel stretch along the back, into the buttock and hips, on your sides as you stretch your arms, and in the front of the legs. Hold the position when you feel the first stretch anywhere, and gradually increase movements as the muscles learn to stretch more comfortably.

Lower Body

Hips – Hip shift:

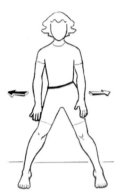

- Stand with your feet comfortably apart: slightly wider than shoulder width apart.
- Feet should be pointing straight ahead.
- Shift or move your hips side to side.
- Keep your legs stay straight and your upper body still. It is just a hip wiggle, back and forth.
- This shift gently stretches the inside and outside areas of the hips.

Hips – Hip shift with knee bend:

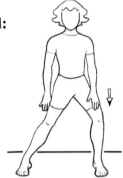

- Stand with your feet comfortably apart: slightly wider than shoulder width apart.
- Bend one leg and shift your weight to that side. Be sure your feet are pointing straight ahead. The knee stays in line with the foot as you bend that leg.
- Your body stays upright. Avoid bending forward.
- This hip shift gently stretches the inside of the straight leg. You will be able to bend the knee further and widen your stance as the muscles begin to learn the stretch.

Hips and Low Back – Crossover:

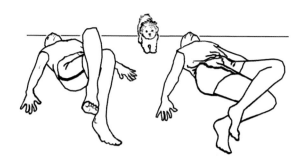

- Lie on the floor with knees bent. Start in a comfortable position, with the feet pulled toward the buttock.
- Cross one leg over the other leg at the knee.
- Use the top leg to gently pull the opposite hip and leg toward the floor. The foot will roll as pull the leg over, but should not kick or shift out to the side. Start with your left leg on top and pull left. You are stretching the right hip and back.
- The shoulders and upper body stay flat, with the arms comfortably near your side.
- Stop the pull when you feel a slight stretch anywhere in the shoulder, side, hip, or leg. A balance of these areas is the goal in the stretch. You will be able to pull the leg closer to the floor as the muscles increase their stretch capability.
- Repeat by stretching the other side: right leg on top, pull right.

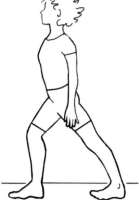

Hips – Standing lunge:

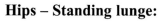

- Stand with one foot forward and the other foot back. The toes should point forward.
- Keep your feet shoulder width apart, not in a straight line, to give better balance.
- Bend your front knee, allowing the hips to move forward. Your knee should not be ahead of the foot as you shift forward.
- Allow the hips to shift with the leg bend while keeping the upper body still; it does not move forward with the hips.
- This stretches the lower abdominal muscles, the front of the hip, and the upper leg.

Hips – Leg off side of bed:

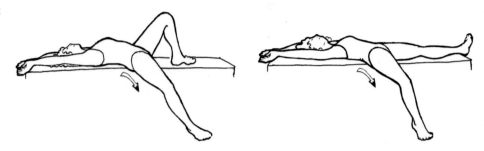

- Lie down near the edge of a bed, a bench, or similar flat surface.
- Bend the leg that is further from the edge of the bed.
- The arms can be near your side or gradually lifted overhead.
- Slowly let the straight leg hang off the side. The tightness in the leg will determine how far the leg lowers. Do not force the movement. The leg will drop further as it loosens.
- As this becomes comfortable, allow both legs to be straight as you let the leg hang off the side of the bed.
- You may feel the stretch through the abdominal area, in the front of the hip, and in the upper leg. Balance among these areas will be attained as the stretch becomes more comfortable.

Hips – End of bed:

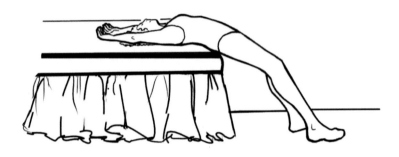

- Sit at the very end of your bed, balanced on the edge, with your feet resting on the floor.
- Slowly lie backward to stretch both sides of the abdominal, hip, and upper leg areas. Slide the feet out to a comfortable position. There should be no discomfort in the lower back.
- If you feel any, slide one foot back towards the bed. If the discomfort continues, stop and do the one leg off the side of the bed until you achieve a better stretch range.

Hips – Sitting lunge:

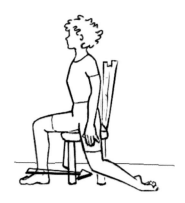

- Select a chair without arms.
- Sit to one side, so one buttock is off the chair.
- Lower the outside leg, reaching backward with the toes tucked under or bent up.
- The knee should not be resting on the floor.
- The upper body stays upright.
- Gradually slide the leg backward, increasing the reach from the hip.
- This stretches the front of the hip and upper leg.

Hips – Kneeling lunge:

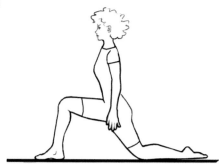

- Kneel on one knee and bend the other leg in front of the body.
- The knee of the top leg should be slightly behind the foot.
- Keep a shoulder-width distance between the knee on the floor and the foot of the opposite leg for better balance.
- Bend or shift the top knee forward while shifting your hips forward.
- Keep the upper body in place; it does not shift forward with the hips.
- This increases hip and upper leg stretch and flexibility.

Back of Upper Leg/Hamstrings – Step stretch:

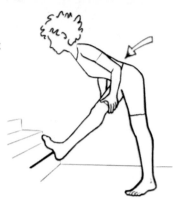

- Stand facing a stair step, chair rung, curb, or something to rest the foot on without the heel's touching the floor.
- Place one foot on the step.
- Keeping the upper body straight, bend forward from the hips, your hands resting on your leg. When you begin to feel a slight stretch or pull in the leg, do not keep bending. Hold that position.
- This position stretches the back of the extended leg. You will be able to bend further and increase the stretch as the leg learns to move to a new, longer position.

Back, Buttock, and Back of Legs – Toe touch:

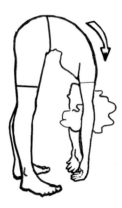

- Stand with the feet comfortably apart, knees straight.
- Lower your head and slowly round the back as you roll down, arms relaxed and reaching toward your feet. Allow your body to hang without tension.
- To return to an upright position, bend your knees and slowly uncurl, lifting your buttock, low-mid-upper back, shoulders, and head in that order.
- You may feel a stretch in the calf muscles as well. This stretch begins to balance the legs and hips.

Back, Buttock, and Back of Legs – Toe touch, version 2; alternate knee bend:

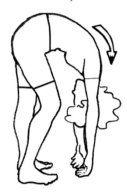

- Repeat the toe touch above, rolling down and reaching toward your feet.
- Slowly bend one knee, keeping the other knee straight.
- This position increases the stretch on the back of the upper leg, the hamstring, and the straight leg.
- Alternate, straightening one knee and bending the opposite one.
- To return to a standing position, bend both knees and slowly roll upward through the buttocks, back, and shoulders, lifting the head last.

Back, Hip, and Legs – Toe touch, version 3; cross leg:

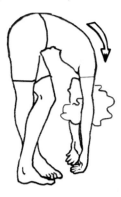

- Cross one leg over the other, starting with the left leg over the right. Your feet should be flat.
- Lower your head, slowly round the back, and roll down as in the toe touch stretches above.
- Turn your hip and upper body to the left, reaching toward your right heel.
- Untwist and bend your knees to slowly roll to an upright position.
- Repeat, crossing the right leg over the left, and rolling down, reaching toward the feet. Twist the hips and upper body to the right this time, reaching for the left heel. Slowly untwist and unroll to an upright standing position.

This stretch increases movement and flexibility on the outside of the hips and legs.

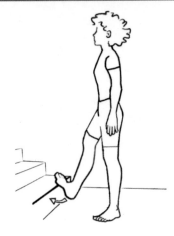

Lower Leg – Calf step stretch:

- Stand facing a stair step, chair rung, curb, or something to rest the foot on without the heel's touching the floor.
- Keeping the upper body upright, place one foot on the step, about level with the ball of the foot.
- Both legs remain straight.
- Slowly lower the heel of the foot on the step. You will feel a stretch or pull in the calf, the back of the lower leg.
- Do not move the heel lower or bounce. When you no longer feel a stretch, gradually increase the distance the heel is lowered.
- The heel should not rest on or touch the floor, as this limits the range of stretch you can attain.

Lower Leg – Full squat:

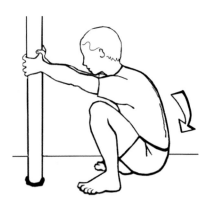

- Grasp something solid with both hands, e.g., doorknobs or a fence post.
- Your feet should be shoulder width apart, toes pointed straight ahead.
- Gradually move into a squat position, holding on for support and balance. Keep your heels flat on the ground.
- The deeper the squat, the greater the stretch on the deep calf muscle (soleus). If you feel any discomfort in the knees, decrease the distance of the squat position.

Ankles – Foot roll:

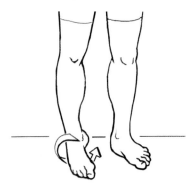

- Standing with your weight on one foot, roll the opposite foot sideways to the outside.
- The rolled foot is not weight bearing. The knee and leg remain straight.
- As the muscles on the outside of the lower leg and ankle increase in their stretch, you will be able to roll the foot so the outside of the foot is on the floor.
- This is a gradual process and should not be forced in any way. Remember, also, it is not weight bearing. The weight is totally on the other leg.
- Attaining this range of movement in the ankle can help prevent many injuries from twisting or rolling the ankle.
- You can practice this stretch while sitting as well. It is important not to allow the leg or knee to move outward at the same time you roll the foot.

Feet – Toes under:

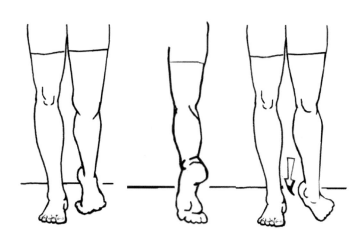

- Standing on both feet, reach one foot behind you.
- Place the toes in a tucked-under position.
- Maintaining that tuck, roll the heel of the foot inward toward the other foot.
- This movement stretches the shin area and the top of the foot.

Feet – Heel raise/on your toes:

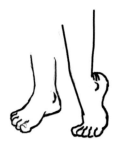

- Standing with your feet shoulder width apart, rise onto the toes of one foot, raising the heel as high as possible.
- The bend in the front of the foot should be at the base of the toes and equal along the joints across the foot. It is common to not bend the big toe equally with the others as it can be stiffer. In that case, add stretching of the toes with your hands when sitting.
- Continue alternately rising onto the toes of one foot, and then the other, being careful to distribute the movement and weight evenly across the front of the foot.
- This heel raise stretches the muscles along the bottom of the foot and eases movement when walking.

The stretches given are intended to form part of the total program presented in this book and are to be used along with all other aspects of the book. They are to be performed as part of teaching muscles a new muscle memory, allowing muscles to function without the tightness that contributes to chronic pain. While an attempt has been made to allow the stretches to be used by everyone, if you have any special needs or concerns, it is important that you consult with your physician before beginning this program.

Appendix 2.
Different Causes of Pain

Chronic pain seems mysterious; it continues to exist no matter how it is addressed. More and more people feel its effects. The table below lists common medical diagnoses: those conditions identified by the medical profession as describing your symptoms and the reason for your pain.

The medical texts *Myofascial Pain and Dysfunction: The Trigger Point Manual, Vols. 1 & 2* document the muscles that are functioning incorrectly and that can cause *the same set of symptoms as the conditions listed in the first column.* It is worth checking out: alleviating the muscle issues and teaching the muscles to function correctly can eliminate the symptoms and pain you experience.

Common Medical Diagnosis	Some of the Muscles Causing the Same Symptoms
Tension (Migraine) Headaches	Sternocleidomastoid (side and front neck muscle) Upper trapezius (upper back and neck muscle) Posterior cervicals (back of neck muscles) Splenii (back of neck muscles) Temporalis (temple muscle)
Acute Stiff Neck	Levator scapulae (shoulder blade to neck muscle) Sternocleidomastoid (side and front neck muscle) Upper trapezius (upper back and neck muscle)
Arthritis of Shoulder	Infraspinatus (rotator cuff shoulder blade muscle)
Subdeltoid (Shoulder) Bursitis	Infraspinatus (rotator cuff shoulder blade muscle) Deltoid (muscle capping the shoulder) Supraspinatus (rotator cuff shoulder blade muscle)
Tennis Elbow (Epicondylitis)	Supinator (elbow muscle) Triceps brachii (back of upper arm)
Carpal Tunnel Syndrome	Scaleni (neck muscles)
Mid-Upper Back Pain	Rectus abdominis (upper portion, abdominal muscle) Levator scapulae (shoulder blade to neck muscle) Rhomboids (shoulder blade to spine muscles)
Low-Back Pain	Rectus abdominis (lower portion, abdominal muscle) Iliopsoas (back and hip muscle)
Hip Pain/Bursitis	Quadratus lumborum (low back and hip muscle) Gluteus maximus and medius (buttock muscles)
Sciatica	Gluteus minimus (deep buttock muscle) Piriformis (deep buttock muscle)
Knee Arthritis	Rectus femoris (quadricep/front of upper leg) Vastus medialis (quadricep/front of upper leg) Vastus lateralis (quadricep/front of upper leg)
Trochanteric (Hip Joint) Bursitis	Vastus lateralis (quadriceps/front of upper leg) Quadratus lumborum (low-back and hip muscle)
Heel Spur	Soleus (deep calf muscle)

Appendix 3.
Contact and Product Resources

Products

Cervical Roll/Pillow: Bed Bath & Beyond   www.bedbathandbeyond.com
Check local telephone listing for stores

Bedding Essentials® Neck Roll Pillow

Foot Rest: Amazon   www.amazon.com
Fellowes: Standard
Rocker
Graphite
Adjustable

Staples   www.staples.com
Check local telephone listing for stores

Fellowes: Model 48121

Heel Lifts: LBM   www.lbmheellifts.com
Phone: 1-800-325-1153

Heel Lift: Height—1/4 inch (most common)
Width (determined by width of the heel of your shoe):
C-0 (narrow), C-1 (wider, most common), or C-2
(wider, for likes of loafer shoes)
Ischial (buttock) Lift: (butt pad to sit on to level hips; use on the
same side of the body as a heel lift)
Thickness—1/4 inch

BML Basics www.bmlbasic.com
Phone: 1-800-643-4751

BML Quality Heel Lift
Width—2 inches for a narrow shoe; 2-1/4
inches for most shoes
Height—7 mm/1/4 inch (most common)
Durometer/Density—D20 (slightly softer) or D40 (most
common)

Ischial (buttock) Lift: (butt pad to sit on to level hips; use on the
same side of the body as a heel lift)
Thickness—1/4 inch

Posture Insoles: Posture Dynamics   www.posturedynamics.com
                              Phone: 1-888-790-4100

ProKinetics®
A full-length shoe insert that is used to address a Dudley Morton's foot, flat arch, or excessive pronation (the foot collapsing inward).

Solemate™
A small insert used to address a Dudley Morton's foot in open-toed shoes, such as sandals with a heel strap.

Wedge Pillows: Dr. Leonard's® Catalog   www.drleonards.com
                             Phone: 1-800-785-0880

Auto Riser: catalog # 81729
This wedge pillow works particularly well when your chair, sofa, or car seat slants backward. Place the narrow end of the pillow at waist level, with your buttocks to the back of the seat. The thicker end fills in the backward slant and holds you upright.

Contact

Nancy Lee Shaw
Myofascial Pain Treatment Center
6417 Loisdale Rd., Suite 308
Springfield, VA 22150
Phone: 703-922-8250
U.S. Country Code: 001-703-922-8250
Email: myoconsult@verizon.net
Skype: nancyls43
www.nancyshawpainclinicandinstitute

Simple Changes
To End
Chronic Pain

Nancy Lee Shaw

Made in the USA
Middletown, DE
11 July 2022

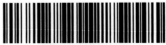